Σmbrace your ΣXCELLENCE

A Psychopharmacology Primer and Mirror to the Soul

"At times our own light goes out and is rekindled by a spark from another person. Each of us has cause to think with deep gratitude of those who have lighted the flame within us."

—Albert Schweitzer
Missionary, Theologian, Nobel Prize Laureate

Diana Rangaves
Santa Rosa Junior College

cognella® | ACADEMIC PUBLISHING

Bassim Hamadeh, CEO and Publisher
Kassie Graves, Director of Acquisitions
Jamie Giganti, Senior Managing Editor
Miguel Macias, Senior Graphic Designer
Jennifer Allen, Acquisitions Editor
Gem Rabanera, Project Editor
Elizabeth Rowe, Licensing Coordinator
Allie Kiekhofer, Chelsey Schmid, and Claire Yee, Interior Designers

Printed in the United States of America

ISBN: 978-1-5165-0414-5 (pbk) / 978-1-5165-0415-2 (br)

cognella® | ACADEMIC PUBLISHING

To my brother

James

ENDOWMENT

One hundred percent of the author's royalties from this publication benefit the Pharmacy Technician Fund at Santa Rosa Junior College Foundation

1501 Mendocino Avenue, Santa Rosa, California 95401

CONTENTS

PREFACE

SIXTY SECONDS WILL PASS AS YOU READ THE FIRST FEW lines of this preface. In those 60 seconds, over **300,000** tweets will enter cyberspace along with numerous Facebook and Instagram posts. In general, many of these informative and visual tidbits live within a tightly networked cyber community; periodically, however, some stir up controversy and enter the worldwide newsfeed.

In another 60 seconds, a healthcare provider will call upon well-honed communication and decision-making skills to make a diagnosis, fill a prescription, or confer with a patient and the patient's family. These real-time decisions impact all involved and depend upon a well-developed, thoughtful, and empathic decision-making approach. Our fast-paced, electronically managed, and information-centric society does not always allow time for measured, thoughtful, reasoned communications and decisions to take shape prior to pressing the send button.

In speeding up our society's collective response time, the powerful and necessary processes needed to support human-centered and reasoned decision-making is neglected. *∑mbrace Your ∑xcellence: A Psychopharmacology Primer and Mirror to the Soul* by Dr. Diana Rangaves invites instructors and students to make room for such decision-making. Readers are invited to combine their interpersonal, empathic, and critical thinking skills to slow down and find the language and knowledge necessary to engage in ethical, thorough, and reflective decision-making, so when they press the send button that articulates their decision (whether through cyberspace or in person), they do so with great confidence that they have made an ethical, empathic, and reasoned decision.

This work-text offers users flexibility in acquiring and refining interpersonal skills to positively impact patient outcomes. Each chapter offers clear objectives, positive affirmations, case studies, opportunities for self-reflection, comprehension checks, and more to help readers develop a cycle of assessment and introspection that informs decision-making that improves quality of care in support of positive patient outcomes. This structure captures what Dr. Martin Luther King, Jr. proposed in his essay "The Purpose of Education." Dr. King wrote, "Intelligence plus character—that is the true goal of education" (drmartinlutherkingjr.com).

This text's comprehensive approach requires students to carefully weave together newly acquired knowledge, their reflections, and social and cultural belief systems to empathetically determine ideal courses of care in any healthcare setting. There is no set script to follow; rather, instructors can choose a specific chapter and select the activities within to develop their students' assessment and reflection skills to fairly and humanely inform their decision-making practices. The wealth of online materials offers instructors and students a healthy and varied collection of supplementary materials to further enhance instruction, exploration, and decision-making.

This book's power and purpose stems from how readers are encouraged to engage in cycle of assessment, self-reflection, and decision-making. Dr. Rangaves weaves together her educational and professional expertise to apprentice readers into this cycle. Her approach emphasizes self-reflection that informs readers' learning and approach to healthcare; in this model, students learn the content that is at the heart of the discipline as well as a "way" of making decisions that has positive impact on patient care.

This approach reaches beyond memorization; it is about engaging in deep, reflective analysis of knowledge, beliefs, assumptions, and biases to delve into the core values required for patient care: interpersonal relations, empathy, informed and reasoned thinking. The work-text encourages students to engage in metacognition to fully understand how they use their knowledge, beliefs, assumptions, and resources to develop decisions. Metacognition, "thinking about one's thinking," invites students to assess their knowledge and views, understand their origins and credibility of them, and then determine what knowledge and views are required in the decision-making process to fully benefit the patient. This process requires that they question what knowledge and beliefs might not positively contribute to the decision-making process, thus, requiring ideological shifts as they revise a decision or prepare to make a new one.

While psychopharmacology is a central topic of this text, so are the topics of decision-making and positive outcomes. Students draw upon the social, personal, cognitive, and knowledge-building dimensions of learning as they engage all parts of this text. These dimensions are central to building mastery in any discipline or practice and depend upon readers' metacognitive processes, helping them maintain awareness of their knowledge, beliefs, assumptions, and how to best analyze situations and problem solve effectively and empathically.

Decisions are not made in isolation. They involve decision-maker(s) and those impacted by the decision. This social nature of decision-making relies upon the same characteristics that describe the social dimension of discipline-specific discourse acquisition: building community; sharing questions, knowledge, and processes; and learning from others. Dr. Rangaves guides readers through the multiple, complex layers of thought through the case studies in this text. Each case is an opportunity to exchange ideas in this real-life situation to surface the multiple views and multiple possibilities that one person alone can rarely see with clarity. Taking the time to exchange ideas and share knowledge allows readers to reexamine their knowledge and beliefs, articulate new discoveries, and synthesize new understandings. Learning requires an openness to accepting a new way of knowing based upon input from others who have valid, pertinent knowledge, which can then cultivate a capacity for empathic interactions with patients.

The personal dimension refers to developing a reader identity, reading confidence and stamina, and metacognitive awareness. In the context of this book, the personal dimension helps students develop awareness of their decision-making identity, confidence about their decisions, stamina for engaging the process fully, and how all of this is dependent upon their metacognitive awareness. Each chapter begins with positive affirmations; each one encourages readers to reflect on current ways of thinking, consider one alternative, and begin the chapter with a new perspective involving positivity and openness.

The cognitive dimension emphasizes the role that problem solving plays in understanding a text; problem solving requires learners to monitor their thinking as they engage with text whether text is conversational, visual, or printed. Metacognitive awareness allows learners to identify when they understand and when they do not understand something within a text. At the moment learners "see" that they do not actually "see" what is in the text, they become problem solvers. This meta view helps learners develop a lens for identifying knowledge and belief systems that might be flawed or impractical and make adjustments.

In the Application sections, readers consider a range of questions requiring them to consider various pieces of information and social and cultural belief systems to develop an approach to a problem. This cognitive awareness first helps learners build the lens and then, over time and with practice, refine how to best use this lens when a problem needs to be solved. Ultimately, this lens helps students trace the thinking behind each decision they make.

The knowledge-building dimension emphasizes the importance of constantly building schema for language, texts, and disciplinary ways of communicating for learners to become increasingly adept at integrating and applying knowledge. Decision-makers must critically assess their own knowledge to ensure it is free of misplaced influences or unanticipated implications. Similarly, in collaborative situations, these decision-makers must also carefully make distinctions between the most pertinent knowledge and the knowledge that is not required within the given context.

As the symbol ∑ in the book title suggests, *∑mbrace Your ∑xcellence: A Psychopharmacology Primer and Mirror to the Soul* provides the sum total of what is required to make empathic decisions that draw upon knowledge, empathy, and self-reflection So, even those decisions that require a response within 60 seconds can be made with confidence when one has practiced and internalized the principles central to empathy-centered inquiry and reasoned decision-making.

Ann Foster, BA, Masters
Professor, Santa Rosa Junior College
California Community Colleges' Success Network (3CSN)
Network and Reading Apprenticeship Coordinator

INTRODUCTION

HELLO AND WELCOME TO *EMBRACE YOUR EXCELLENCE—A Psychopharmacology Primer and Mirror to the Soul.* First, I would like to start by saying thank you. Thank you for choosing to teach your students the critical skills needed.

In recent years, more focus has been placed on healthcare quality and achieving positive patient outcomes. With our knowledge, skills, and accessibility, we are uniquely positioned to be drivers of quality.

By taking the time to teach your students these skills, you are preparing them for careers in this evolving healthcare model.

As a participant in this textbook, you have access to web-based platforms, MTM cases, presentations, implementation guides, and training materials. You can use as few or as many of these resources as you would like.

The education and preparation of our academic competencies incorporate innovative teaching strategies so enhanced that we become methodical, self-directed, critical thinkers.

Critical thinking for decision-making is the ability to think in a systematic and logical manner with openness to question and reflect on the reasoning process used to ensure safety and quality. (Heaslip)

Escape into Excellence—A Psychopharmacology Primer and Mirror to the Soul provides a comprehensive integration of knowledge, comprehension, application, analysis, synthesis, and evaluation via engaging case scenarios, text exercises, interactive retention activities, video, and reading links.

The course instructor and/or students can collaboratively self-select content and activities to allow for the maximum degree of creativity and individual flexibility. In essence, pieces from each module can be woven into a unique tapestry enhancing the personalized learning experience.

Each module features cohesive objectives and key terms, multicultural case illustrations, assimilated development and consequences of the paradigm, student centered learning activities, and text enquiries. These may be coupled with instructor-generated ancillaries.

The instructor, as guide, side-by-side with students, will build a rich diverse language of knowledge and competencies.

The modules feature an extensive variety of hands-on materials for the individual, small group, and larger class endeavor, which develops knowledge and checks for understanding.

Instructors may freely conduct students to cooperate, interrelate, and create fresh thought network links by writing directly in the text.

Learning opportunities and reading strategies are incorporated to capture the process. Interactive Keywords, Think-Aloud, Think-Pair-Share, Talking to the Text, Questions, Mapping, in pairs, groups, and as individuals create a unique relationship with the material.

Navigation of the text structures includes:

- Responding to questions that targeting "thinking about thinking."
- Readings that deepen understanding.
- Analyses which expand concepts.
- Anonymous cases which embed and illustrate modeling.
- Visual images that support meaningful practice.
- Applications which capture the skills and ability to express oneself.

These modules are an integral series of elements in the progression of enacting confidence and substance in "seeing" the significance of a bigger picture.

VISUAL IMAGE STRUCTURES

Readers will encounter the following icons throughout each chapter to demarcate different sections.

Chapter Objectives

Student learning outcomes are the effects and objectives of acquiring the knowledge.

Positive Affirmations

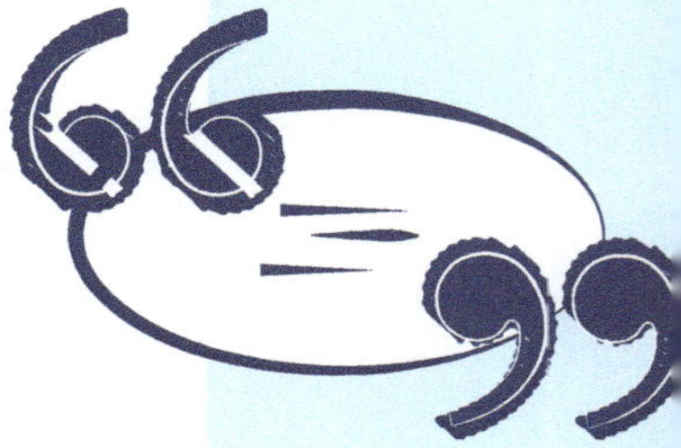

A transitional quote relevant to the chapter topic. It is the voyage from one place of thought to another, as in Think-Aloud.

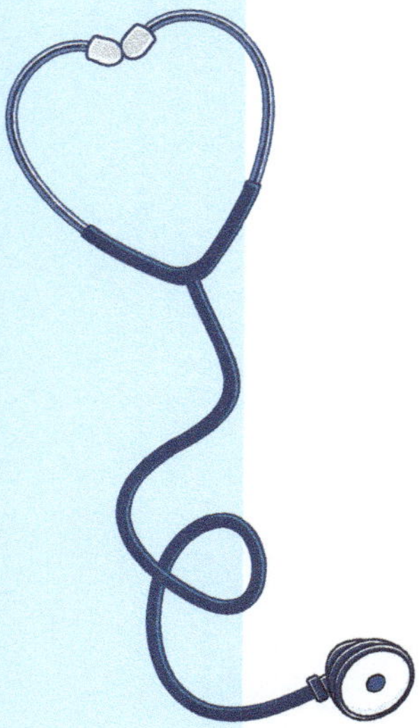

Pharmacology

Knowledge-based concepts, instruction, ideas, and principles. This section consists of readings that deepen understanding.

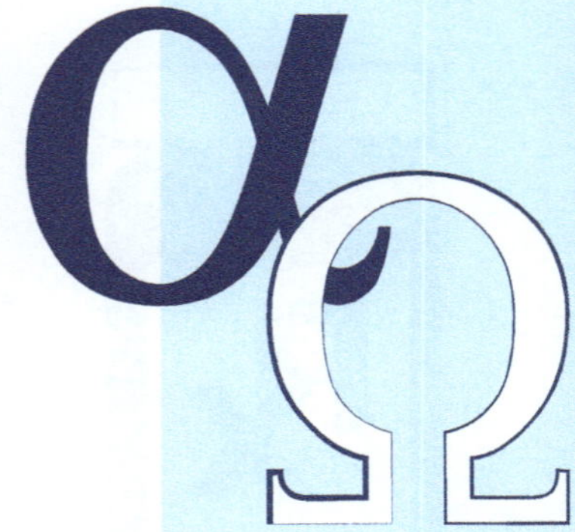

Alpha Omega

This icon indicates cases of addiction, recovery, and advocacy. In this section, anonymous cases are shared to embed and illustrate modeling: Think-Pair-Share.

Critical Thinking

A portrayal paradigm of "What do you see?" This section consists of applications which capture the skills and ability to express oneself: Talking to the Text.

WISH: Wise Inner Soul Harmony.

This section contains web links to visual images that support meaningful practice in audio and video in animation content form.

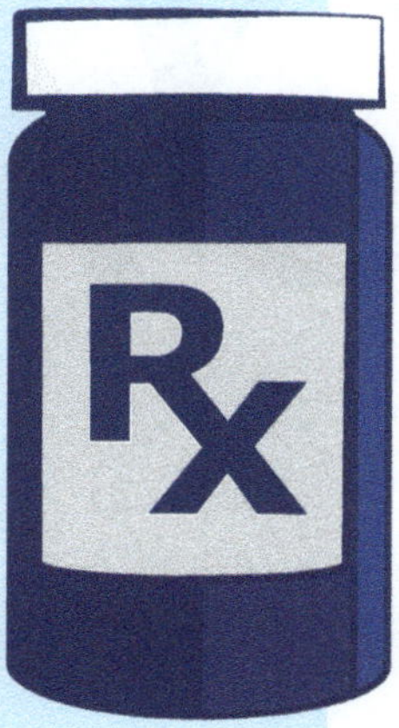

Drug Sandbox

Important vocabulary words to know!

Community Connections

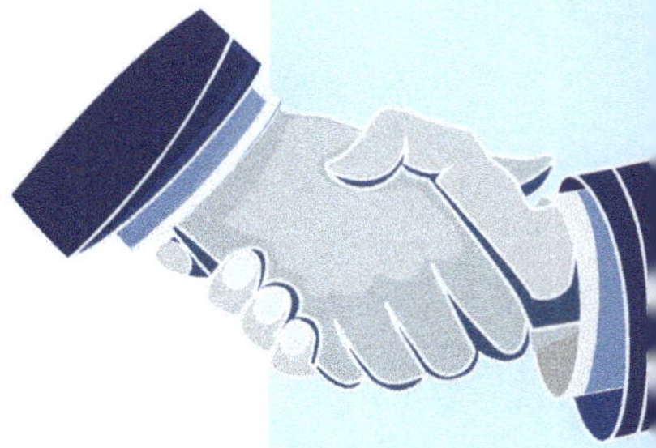

Recovery model of programs and modalities analyses which expand concepts.

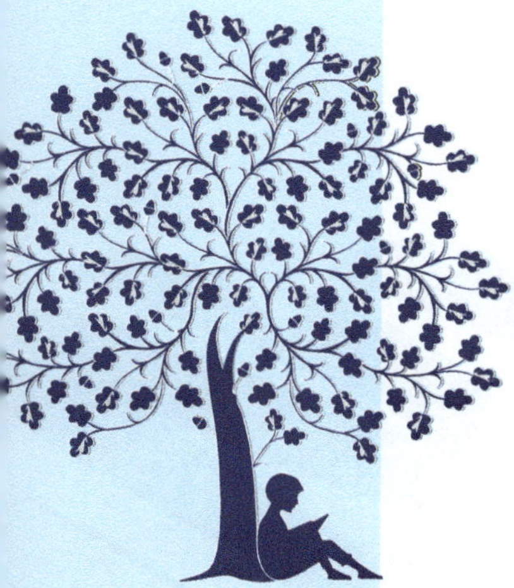

End of Chapter Review Questions

Application

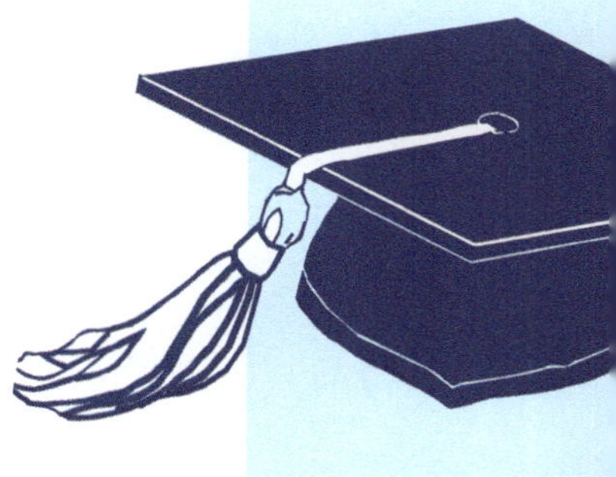

Assessments of usage and relevance. This section provides end of chapter discussion questions and asks readers to respond to questions that target "thinking about thinking."

CHAPTER ONE

THE OPENING

Chapter Objectives

1. Differentiate responsibilities of thinking and reactivity.
2. Interpret and apply the relabel, refocus, reattribute, and revalue technique of mindfulness.
3. Differentiate among the major areas of pharmacology.
4. Describe the nervous system, neurotransmitters, agonist, and antagonist.
5. Identify the terms of basic pharmacology, substance abuse and misuse, drug names, classifications, the Controlled Substances Act, and the FDA Pregnancy Safety Categories.

Positive Affirmations

"In a gentle way, you can shake the world."

—Gandhi

"Persistence is what makes the impossible possible, the possible likely, and the likely definite"

—Robert Half

"We cannot solve problems with the same mindset that we use to create them. One does not change a system by criticizing it; one finds ways to make the old model obsolete."

—Albert Einstein

A Beginning

"On January 27 at approximately 4:30 p.m., I was in front of the DMV with a weapon and methamphetamine on my person. It had been a long two weeks as I looked for the person who had shot my friend to death. Trying to take care of errands while I launched my own manhunt had ill effects when mixed with dope. Eventually, I ended up getting arrested because, to no one's surprise, the authorities had been waiting to 'ask me some questions.' Before we examine what came of this eventful afternoon, perhaps a bit of background is in order.

"Starting around the year 2000, I was involved in a lifestyle that wasn't appealing to a lot of people. Between the gangs and drugs, it was easy to see why this was an acquired lifestyle. As the years went on, I found myself getting more arrogant and cocky about having never been caught and watching everybody else who had. As the drugs and guns increased, so did my warped point of view of how the world runs and what it takes to survive in it. Things got more complicated as the years went along as well as more dangerous. It culminated with my friend getting killed and me getting arrested in connection to everything that surrounded it.

"Fast-forward to September, and I am released from jail after serving the time the authorities saw fit. During my time in jail, I questioned why we exist to begin with. What is it about this life that makes us want to continue, and is there a reason that we are even capable of asking such questions? I started to investigate heavily all the different types of worldviews, views that ranged from atheism, to agnosticism, Christianity, Islam, Hinduism, New Age, and so on. I believed God had a purpose in allowing these events to happen. So I dedicated myself to that cause and helping people see that their life matters, and there is a better way to live life by helping others out of the trouble they are in. Maybe it would open the door to a healthier understanding of the world that we live in."—Anonymous

"In a gentle way, one can shake the world," can be a prologue to understanding the brain, behaviors, and accompanying release of neurotransmitters.

Psychotropic medications stem from the root "trop," meaning to turn toward, to change position, to face. The word integrity has its roots in the Latin word "integritatem," meaning "soundness" or "wholeness" of mind. The ultimate goal of Jungian psychoanalysis is for one to become "whole" from fragmented parts of the personality; some of these aspects of self are buried in the unconscious or part of one's "shadow." The shadow contains all the disassociated parts of one's personality and implies that one is unaware of the contents of this part of the psyche.

Integrity is linked to the words "integral" or "integrated" and means a unified whole. When one has a more integrated personality, a person would ideally be connected to all parts of his or her psyche; thus, all parts of his or her physical self and all parts of his or her spiritual self-making become a powerful unified functioning self in the world. The person would naturally feel more connected to the universe and see him or herself as an integral part of it; any harm to the outer world means harm to the inner.

When one is dishonest or acts in a way that is harmful to another person, the potential for an integrated bond is broken. Unethical or intentionally harmful acts cause a "divide" within a person. It would seem logical that one has to internally justify causing harm so that the divide within resulting from the reality of such behavior further deepens. This is why it is so important to at least try to act with integrity in all that we do so as to keep ourselves as whole and as integrated as possible.

The brain changes; it is neuroplastic! Thoughts are just thoughts. Keep flexibility as a companion. Dr. Jeffrey Schwartz's Four Steps: "Relabel, Reattribute, Refocus, and Revalue" REMAIN Neutral.

RELABEL them; they can be false signals.

REATTRIBUTE them; they are not real. It is only the brain talking, a neural glitch. The brain is stuck in a "worry circuit." Now have the mind act back on the brain. Stand outside your brain as the watcher, the witness, the bystander. Investigate the causes of the thought; reflect and learn from the process. By putting the spotlight on mindful attention, you can engage plasticity and attention and enable change.

REFOCUS; false signals have no power. Take the time and work to push yourself cognitively to alter the brain map. Have the drive and willingness to leave your comfort zone and "dance a new dance." It is an acquired skill. We must work to maintain our figures! We must work to maintain our brain.

REVALUE; remember, false signals have no power. Fear has no power, it is simply False Evidence Appearing Real.

Pharmacology

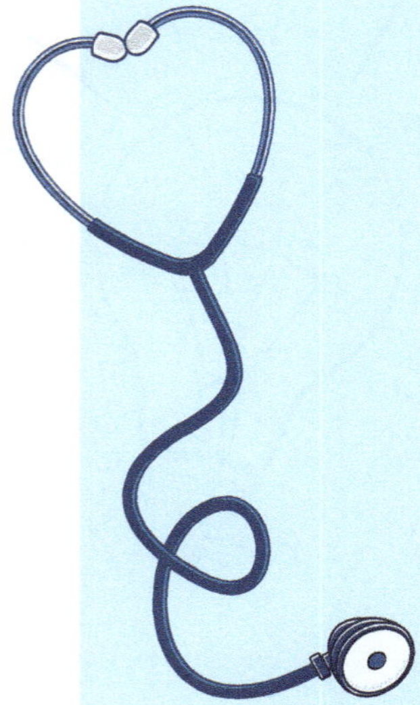

WELCOME to PHARMACOLOGY and PSYCHOPHARMACOLOGY!

MAJOR AREAS OF PHARMACOLOGY

- **Pharmacology:** A science that studies the effects of drugs within a living system.
- **Toxicology:** Concerned with the harmful effects of drugs
- **Pharmacy:** The study of preparing and dispensing medications and a place.
- **Pharmacotherapeutics:** How drugs are used in the treatment of disease.
- **Pharmacodynamics:** How a drug behaves in the body system.
- **Pharmacokinetics:** How a drug moves through the body system.

Alpha Omega

αΩ

"I enter this new time with the understanding that I am making a fresh start. I begin by discarding thoughts, attitudes, and habits that are not compatible with an excellent life. I let go of whatever caused past discouragement, disappointment, or disagreement. I know that seemingly negative outcomes are desires or goals that are yet to be fulfilled. I am open and receptive to new ideas, activities, and relationships.

"Each day, I can follow a fresh plan of fulfillment. I act on divine ideas that I receive as inspiration. These ideas flow through wholesome, positive thoughts. As I use creative thinking to build upon divine ideas, my activities become more dynamic and my abilities are enhanced. Therefore, I enter this new time with optimism, joy and enthusiasm." —Anonymous

Critical Thinking

FOCUS ON THE OBJECTIVE

If the thoughts you are thinking are not giving you that "good feeling," then think about something else that will make you feel good in that moment. Observe your thoughts and ideas consistently throughout the day. Sometimes this may not be as easy as you think if you are stuck in a "destructive" train of thought, and your brain chemicals are getting fired up and forming "anxiety or anger" thoughts. Anxiety, fear, and anger patterns can be interrupted by focusing on something else. This will dissipate the rush of chemicals that are making you feel bad. Immediately, then, go back to picturing scenes/remembering things/imagining, planning stuff that makes you feel good.

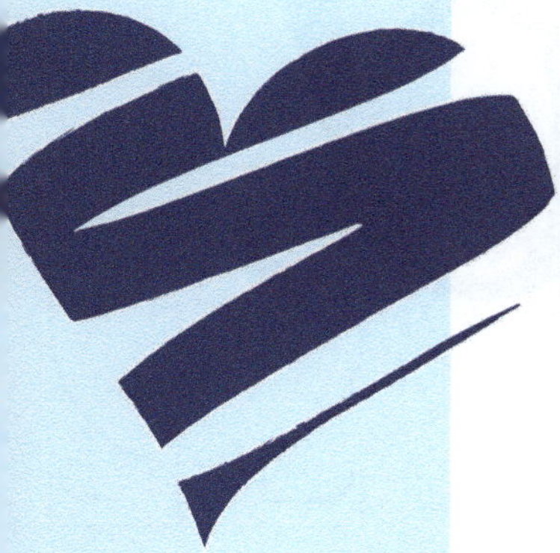

WISH

Everything You Think You Know About Addiction TED Talk:

https://www.youtube.com/watch?v=PY9DcIMGxMs&feature=youtu.be

What is Addiction:

https://www.youtube.com/watch?v=T5sOh4gKPIg&feature=youtu.be

The Power of Addiction and the Addiction of Power:

https://www.youtube.com/watch?v=66cYcSak6nE&feature=youtu.be

Spiders on Drugs:

https://www.youtube.com/watch?time_continue=3&v=sHzdsFiBbFc

Ten Most Addictive Drugs:

https://www.youtube.com/watch?v=Edi3ta0lkAA

Getting Stupid: How Drugs Damage the Brain:

http://www.nhs.uk/Livewell/drugs/Pages/Dodrugsdamagebrain.aspx

Human Body: How the Central Nervous System Works:

https://www.youtube.com/watch?v=1-wsFt2UmoM

Neuron Neurotransmitters:

https://www.youtube.com/watch?v=p5zFgT4aofA

Agonists and Antagonists:

http://www.interactive-biology.com/1641/agonists-and-antagonists-episode-18/

Teenage Star to Addicted and Homeless:

http://www.youtube.com/watch?v=KiYFc6Zpbjo

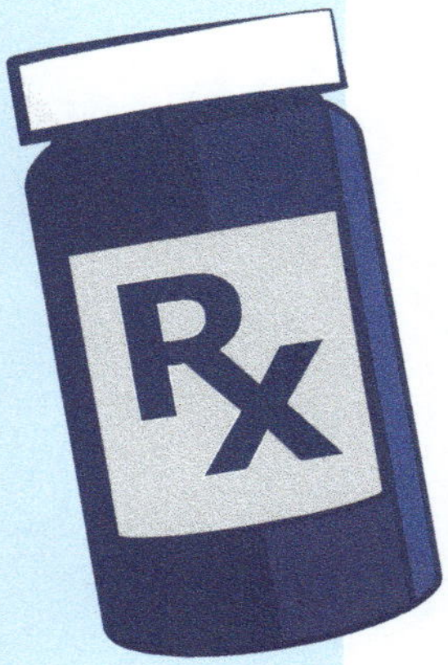

Drug Sandbox

BASIC TERMINOLOGY

Adverse Effect
Agonist
Antagonist
Chemical Name
Contraindications
Dose
Drug
Drug Indication
Generic Name

Mechanism of Action
Over-the-Counter (OTC)
Pharmacology
Prescription Drug
Receptor
Side Effect
Site of Action
Trade Name
Placebo

SUBSTANCE MISUSE AND ABUSE TERMS

Drug Misuse
Substance Abuse

Drug Abuse
Physical Dependence

Psychological Dependence
Addiction
Illicit Drugs
Tolerance

DRUG NAMES AND CLASSIFICATIONS

Atomic (Molecular) Composition
Chemical Name
Structural Formula
Nonproprietary Name (Generic)
Stems and Classes
Therapeutic Class
Proprietary Name
NDC #

CONTROLLED SUBSTANCES ACT

Schedule I (Heroin)
Schedule II (Methadone)
Schedule III (Valium®)
Schedule IV (Alprazolam)
Schedule V (Lomotil®)

FDA PREGNANCY SAFETY CATEGORIES

Category A: Adequate studies indicate no risk to the fetus in the first trimester and no evidence of risk in later trimesters.

Category B: Animal reproduction studies have not demonstrated a risk to fetus; no well-controlled human studies.

Category C: Animal studies report adverse effect on fetus; no human studies; no benefit/risk assessments.

Category D: There is evidence of human fetal risk, but the potential benefits from the use of the drug may be acceptable if safer drugs are not available or ineffective.

Category X: Studies in animal or humans demonstrate fetal abnormalities or adverse reaction reports indicating fetal risk. Risk outweighs any benefit. These drugs should not be used in pregnant women.

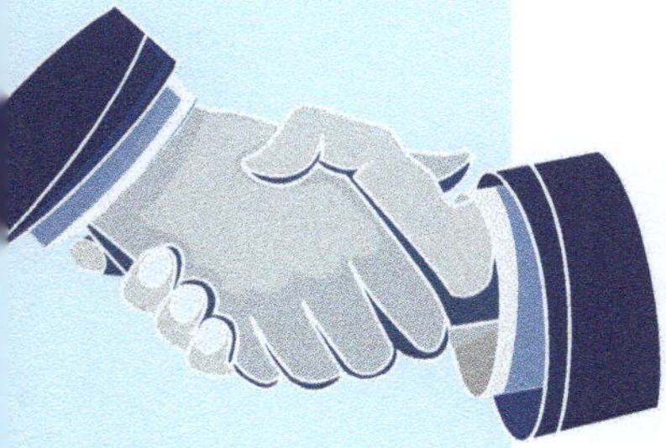

Community Connections

COGNITIVE BEHAVIORAL THERAPY

> "The definition of insanity is doing the same thing over and over again and expecting different results."
>
> —Albert Einstein.

Every addict could most likely relate to this logic. No one wants to be addicted to drugs, alcohol, or behaviors, but it is very difficult to change patterns of thinking or behavior.

A basic explanation of Cognitive Behavioral Therapy, or CBT, is to recondition one's thoughts brought on by emotions to aide in changing behaviors. Behavioral patterns of humans generally come from having a feeling, deciding on a thought about that feeling, and then acting out the observable behavior. "This technique acknowledges that there may be behaviors that cannot be controlled through rational thought but rather emerge based on prior conditioning from the environment and other external and/or internal stimuli" (National Institute).

Cognitive behavioral therapy is all based around our negative thoughts and how they can control our behaviors. A majority of our negative thoughts are imbedded in us from our childhood. The process encourages the breakdown of thoughts, feelings, and behaviors that trap us in a negative cycle and teaches skills and strategies that can be applied in the coping of everyday life.

Specific techniques include exploring the positive and negative consequences of continued behaviors, drug use and patterns, using self-monitoring to recognize cravings early, identifying situations that might put one at risk for use, and then developing strategies for coping with cravings and avoiding those high-risk situations (Matano).

CBT had its origin in the 1960s with William Beck; however, there are others who paved the way for Cognitive Behavioral Therapy. According to the National Alliance of Cognitive-Behavioral Therapists, it was Dr. Albert Ellis with his RET (Rational Emotive Therapy) who started the groundwork for CBT in the 1950s. His development of RET was in response to a dissatisfaction with the nature of psychoanalysis. In the 1960s, Dr. Maxie Maultsby introduced client rational self-counseling and therapeutic homework for the clients. Dr. Alfred Adler (psychotherapist) has been given credit as most influential to the development of RET from which CBT arose. "I am convinced that a person's behavior springs from his ideas."(Adler) The psychoanalytic aspect of therapy has been around for many years and continues to contribute to mental health and addiction treatment.

According to the Royal College of Psychiatrists, there are five areas in which the CBT process is addressed: First, there is a situation; something that is going on in the person's life that he or she is having a difficult time dealing with. Second comes thoughts. What goes on in his or her mind when this situation is brought up? Third are emotions. What types of feelings arise when thinking about the situation? This can lead to the fourth area of physical feelings. There can be physical consequences to stress and overthinking things that can cause actual physical responses in the body. The fifth area is actions. What will the patient do when the previous four areas are taken into account? Will it be a behavior that is beneficial or negative? Will it be a repeated pattern or a one-time thing?

For example, when Alice feels sad she associates that feeling with vulnerability and weakness because she was taught to never show other people that she is sad. So, Alice bottles up her sadness time and time again until she explodes with uncontrollable sobbing over something irrelevant. These outbursts leave her depressed and unmotivated, so she starts using cocaine to go about her daily living. Her life starts to become unmanageable. She is continuously tardy and behind at work. Her bills are left unpaid, and she begins to lose possessions and friends. She is irrational, angry, and depressed. She decides to see a therapist where she begins CBT.

Through intensive processing with her therapist, together they identify the association Alice has with showing emotions. CBT takes the thought that "showing feelings makes me a vulnerable and weak person," and Alice has to repeatedly replace the thought with "showing my feelings makes me human; it is my authentic self. When I hide my feelings, I am denying my true self." Over time, Alice starts to believe the new thought more and more. She takes steps in showing emotions around people she trusts. She starts to see improved functioning with fewer outbursts. As she continues her CBT, she no longer believes that she is weak or vulnerable if she shows emotions. She accepts herself and starts to love herself more. She uses less and less drugs. She is doing better at work and rebuilding relationships.

It takes Alice a long time to start to see changes in her behavior. She has to be conscious of her thought patterns and make an effort to combat the ones that negatively affect her behavior. She is committed to change and works closely with her therapist. A client must be willing to do some internal processing, seek out supportive reading material, and try new ways of thinking in order to see results. If a client is coming to therapy prompted by criminal justice system, he or she may not have a desire or be capable of participating in his or her treatment.

CBT differs from many other types of psychotherapies because sessions have a structure rather than the person talking freely about whatever comes to mind. The client meets the therapist to describe specific problems, and they set goals they want to work towards. It has been concluded that CBT is one of the most effective interventions. "According to the National Institute on Drug Abuse, more than 24 randomized controlled trials have been conducted among users of tobacco, alcohol, cocaine, marijuana, opiates, and other types of substances, making cognitive-behavioral treatments one of the more frequently evaluated psychosocial approaches to treat substance use disorders" (McHugh).

Cognitive Behavioral Therapy is a treatment modality used in a wide range of mental illnesses; however, some clients with more severe mental illness may not be well enough to participate in the treatment. CBT cannot help cure the hallucinations of a schizophrenic. Some may have improved abilities to recognize that they are hallucinating, and some may not be able differentiate. CBT is often paired with antidepressant and antipsychotic medications to treat the chemical imbalances. Most of the irrational beliefs we form come from childhood experience and are programmed reactions; if a client doesn't continue to reassess, he or she can fall right back into old behaviors.

More recently, CBT has had successful results in the process of addiction treatment. In terms of treatment for addiction and relapse, CBT was first used to help alcoholics recover. Today, CBT has been adapted and is used in treatment for other substances including cocaine, methamphetamine, marijuana, and nicotine addiction. As addiction treatment becomes more focused on long-term recovery, CBT is being used more frequently to compliment the acute specialty care phase. CBT has been successful in enabling many individuals to actually avoid relapsing or to shorten the length of time of a relapse. Therapy strategies include clients participating in identifying problematic behaviors and connecting these behaviors to their addictions.

The concept that the development of maladaptive behavioral patterns like substance abuse can be created by certain learning processes plays an important role in these behaviors (Caroll). New skills are looked at and applied to help the individual stop relapsing or using in the first place. Other problematic behaviors that co-occur with addiction are addressed, as well. CBT methods use this psychotherapy technique to establish behavioral modifications and verbal interventions. As clients identify habitual thinking and patterns, they can develop new behaviors that help them stay away from the substance they are struggling with. These new tools also assist the person in the area of "changing" old behaviors and habits into positive outcomes.

The first step into any type of treatment modality is to stop the using and abusing behaviors. With this first step comes the realization that relearning behaviors can be frustrating and stressful. The process of recovery starts with identifying the problem, being willing to change and look for solutions, and then rebuilding a strong personal foundation to carry one forward.

Cognitive Behavioral Therapy addresses many of these issues for the willing and dedicated participant; the results can be many, with few side effects or expense of medications. Clients can lead more productive lives and have better personal relationships. They can overcome many horrific experiences that shaped a negative outlook or low self-esteem. Clients can maintain their own form of inner processing and self-perception long after the CBT sessions have ended. CBT is a way to help clients change their life for the better. It provides emotional, social, and physical wellness for the long term.

End Of Chapter Review Questions

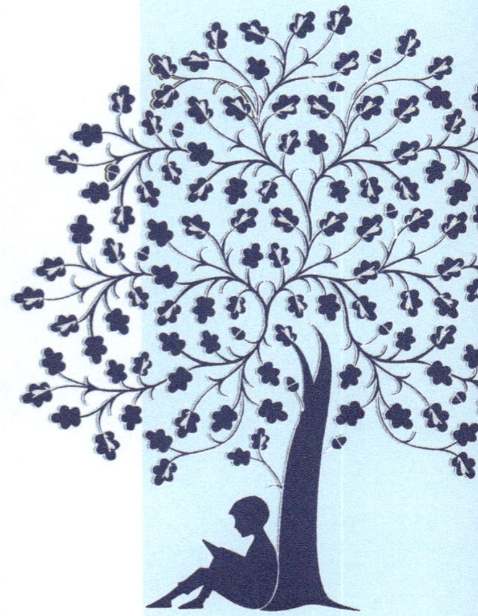

Select the letter that matches the following words with their appropriate meanings:

1.	Generic	a.	Inactive substance with no treatment value
2.	Receptor	b.	Name of an agent given by the manufacturer
3.	Agonists	c.	Drugs which block cellular response
4.	Placebo	d.	Drugs which exert similar actions to the body own response
5.	Antagonists	e.	Molecule on the surface or within a cell that causes cellular effect

Indicate if the following statements are true (A) or false (B):

6. State law divides controlled substances into five schedules according to their drug equivalence, safety, and effectiveness.

7. Safety categories for use during pregnancy are based on all available information and tests on pregnant women.

Multiple Choices: Select the best answer from the choices given:

8. FDA pregnancy categories are:
    a. A, B, C, D, X
    b. CI, CII, CIII, CIV, CV
    c. Class 1, Class 2, Class 3
    d. Phase I, Phase II, Phase III, Phase IV

9. Which of the following drug schedules has no acceptable medical use in the US.?
    a. Schedule I, C-I
    b. Schedule II, C-II
    c. Schedule III, C-III
    d. Schedule IV, C-IV
    e. Schedule V, C-V

10. A patient has been on high doses of OxyContin for cancer pain for six months. She does not experience euphoria when taking the prescribed dosage and has no need or desire to take increasing doses or commit illegal behaviors. She continues to work and contribute to the community. Therefore, she is most likely to be __________ to the OxyContin.
    a. Dependent
    b. Addicted
    c. Tolerant
    d. Inducted

Applications: Assessment of Usage and Relevance

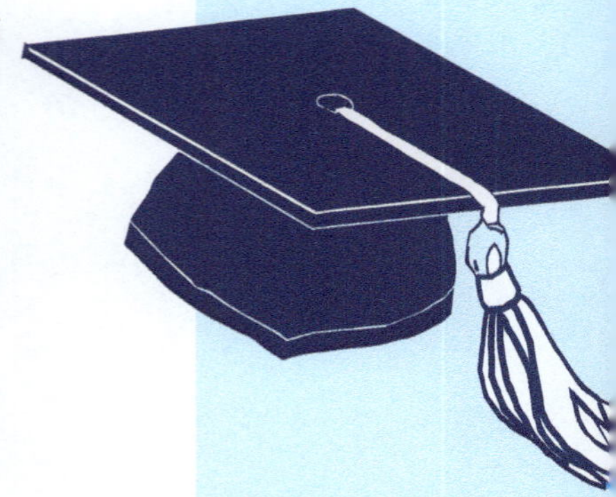

Use the Internet to research and collect information with the questions below as a guide. Compare your findings in class.

1. Explain the practical and theoretical issues surrounding drug classification.

2. Describe seven ways drugs may be classified.

3. Explain four principles of psychoactive drug effects.

4. Explain the many manifestations of tolerance.

5. Can someone be harmed by a dosage of a drug to which tolerance has been developed? How?

KEY

1. B	4. A	7. B	10. A
2. E	5. C	8. A	
3. D	6. B*	9. A	

*according to their level of addiction potential and accepted medical use

REFERENCES

Cognitive Behavioral Therapy: The Four Steps—Dr. Jeffrey Schwartz's Four Steps. Relabel, Reattribute, Refocus, Revalue, REMAIN Neutral: http://hope4ocd.com/foursteps.php.

"Cognitive-Behavioral Therapy (Alcohol, Marijuana, Cocaine, Methamphetamine, Nicotine)." National Institute of Drug Abuse. N.p., Dec. 2012. Web. 2 Oct. 2015. https://www.drugabuse.gov/publications/principles-drug-addiction-treatment-research-based-guide-third-edition/evidence-based-approaches-to-drug-addiction-treatment/behavioral.

Kennard, Jerry. "Benefits and Limitations of Cognitive Behavioral Therapy (CBT) for Treating Anxiety. http://www.healthcentral.com/anxiety/c/4182/165578/benefits-limitations-treating/#sthash.sfD6DqnG.dpuf."

Health Central. N.p., 6 Jan. 2014. Web. 4 Oct. 2015. http://www.healthcentral.com/anxiety/c/4182/165578/benefits-limitations-treating/.

"Behavior Therapy for Alcoholics." About Health. n.p., 28 Nov. 2014. Web. 5 Oct. 2015. http://alcoholism.about.com/od/relapse/a/cbt.htm.

Center for Substance Abuse Treatment. Substance Abuse Treatment: Group Therapy. Rockville (MD): Substance Abuse and Mental Health Services Administration (US); 2005. (Treatment Improvement Protocol [TIP] Series, No. 41.) 2 Types of Groups Commonly Used in Substance Abuse Treatment. Available from: http://www.ncbi.nlm.nih.gov/books/NBK64214/.

Center for Substance Abuse Treatment. Substance Abuse Treatment for Adults in the Criminal Justice System. Rockville (MD): Substance Abuse and Mental Health Services Administration (US). 2005. (Treatment Improvement Protocol (TIP) Series, No. 44.) 5 Major Treatment Issues and Approaches. Available from: http://www.ncbi.nlm.nih.gov/books/NBK64124/.

CBT or Psychodynamic Therapy (n.d.). Retrieved October 4, 2015, from http://cbtvs-psychodynamic.com/ProsandCons.html.

Cognitive Behavior Therapy for Substance Abuse. (n.d.). Retrieved October 4, 2015, from http://www.beckinstitute.org/cbt-for-substance-abuse/.

Matano, R. A., Yalom, I. D., and Schwartz, K. Interactive group therapy for substance abusers. In: Spira, J. L., ed. Group Therapy for Medically Ill Patients. New York: Guilford Press, 1997. pp. 296–325.

McHugh, R. K., Hearon, B. A., and Otto, M. W. (2010). Cognitive-Behavioral Therapy for Substance Use Disorders. The Psychiatric Clinics of North America, 33(3), 511–525. http://doi.org/10.1016/j.psc.2010.04.012.

Prochaska, J., DiClemente, C., Norcross, J., (1992). In search of how people change. Applications to addictive behaviors. Am Psychol 47:1102.

What is Cognitive-Behavioral Therapy? (n.d.). Retrieved October 5, 2015, from http://www.nacbt.org/whatiscbt.htm.

www.nhs.uk/conditions/cognitive-behavioral-therapy/Pages/Advantages.aspx.

www.psychcentral.com/lib/in-depth-congitive-behavioral-therapy/3/3.

www.counseling-diretory.org.uk/congitive-behavioral-therapy.html#iscbteffective.

Carroll, K. M., and Onken, L. S. Behavioral therapies for drug abuse. The American Journal of Psychiatry 168(8): 1452–1460, 2005.

"How CBT Can Help Addiction Treatment Be More Recovery-Oriented." Alcoholism & Drug Abuse Weekly 24.31 (2012): 1–3. CINAHL Complete. Web. 13 Sept. 2015. www.addictions.com/cognitive-behavioral.

CHAPTER TWO

THE BODY

Chapter Objectives

1. Differentiate aspects of the pharmacokinetics.
2. Express and apply the elements of pharmacodynamics.
3. Differentiate among the types of drug action.
4. Distinguish the primary central nervous system neurotransmitters.
5. Identify the principles of serum concentration and effect terms.

Positive Affirmations

> "The greater danger for most of us lies not setting our aim too high and falling short; but in setting our aim too low and achieving our mark."
>
> —Michelangelo

Pharmacology

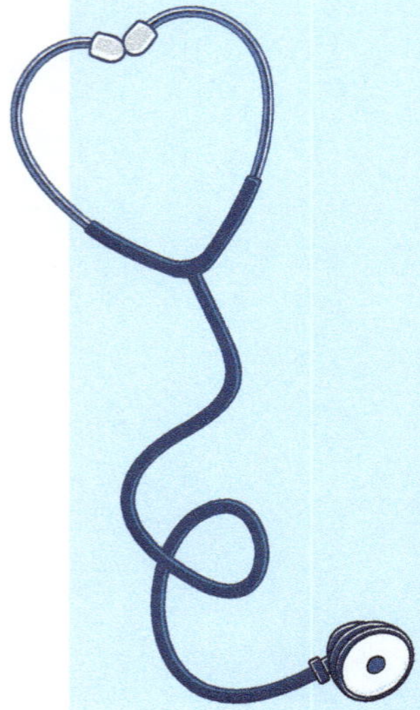

How do drugs work? How do they "know" to go from one's stomach to our head and not the foot?

In basic biopharmaceutics, the objective of drug therapy is to deliver the right drug, in the right concentration, to the right site of action, and at the right time to produce the desired effect (and, of course, to the right patient!).

THE EFFECTS of DRUGS OCCUR THROUGH SEVERAL TYPES of DRUG ACTION. THEY ARE:

- React physically with receptors
- React chemically with nonspecific membrane lipids
- Modify metabolic activity and enzyme systems
- Have an osmotic effect: no direct action on cell
- Interfere with normal cell function
- Modify ion channels
- Modify creation, release, or control of neurotransmitters or hormones

Receptors are cellular material at the site of action that are responsible for the brain chemistry behind primary motor and thoughts. Neurotransmitters bind to a specific receptor in a "lock and key" process. One needs to fit the other in order to exert any effect. The effect can be as an agonist (similar) or antagonist (blocker). These chemical messengers are responsible for the mechanism of drug action, or how a drug knows to go to the foot or head!

THE PRIMARY CENTRAL NERVOUS SYSTEM (CNS) NEUROTRANSMITTERS ARE:

- Acetylcholine (Ach)
- Aspartate
- Dopamine (DA)
- GABA (inhibitory neurotransmitter)
- Glutamate (excitatory neurotransmitter)
- Norepinephrine (NE)
- Serotonin (5-HT)

PHARMACOKINETICS

There `are multiple phases of drug activity. Pharmacokinetics is the action of drugs in the body over a period of time, or how a drug MOVES through the body.

These elements are ADME:
Absorption
Distribution
Metabolism
Elimination

What is Half-life? What do you think this means?

- The time taken for the drug concentration to decline by 50%.
- The time taken for 50% of the drug to be eliminated.
- The time taken for the drug concentration to fall to half the original value.

OR

- The time taken for the drug concentration to fall to half the original value.

The answers are!

After four half-lives, elimination is 94% complete.
After seven half-lives, elimination is 99% complete
After one half-life, elimination is___? complete. (Answer: 50%)

PHARMACODYNAMICS

Pharmacodynamics is how a drug behaves. It can be either beneficial or toxic. Drugs bind to a receptor with differing affinity. They can exert an agonist effect or an antagonist effect. Drug interactions occur when the actions of one drug are affected by another drug. These include additive effects, summation, synergism, and antagonism.

Anticholinergic Side Effects

- Dry mouth
- Blurred vision
- Rapid heart rate (tachycardia)
- Urine retention
- Constipation
- Confusion and memory impairment
- Kidneys

Harmful Responses/Adverse Effects

- CNS effects
- Hepatotoxicity
- Hypersensitivity or allergy
- GI effects
- Nephrotoxicity
- Hematological effects
- Drug dependence
- Teratogenicity
- Carcinogenicity
- Idiosyncrasy

Drug Use Definitions

- Dependence: State in which the body has adapted physiologically and psychologically
- Addiction: Need to take/do something to attain effects with a decrease functioning
- Abuse: Purposeful drug amounts taken for other than prescribed use
- Tolerance: Decrease in response to drug effect after continued administration

Alpha Omega

"Why I am here studying to become a counselor is a long story, but the story certainly starts with my childhood. I was born into a family of educators, French/German/Irish Catholic, and alcoholism. My father, my great grandfather, my aunts and uncles, my brothers, and cousins; this coupled with mental illness: bipolar and depression. I now know that my dad was self-medicating and understand how much he was suffering. I went to Alateen in high school. In my 30s I worked the steps in Love Addicts Anonymous. The 12 Steps saved my life; so did God. I tried to kill myself twice, and both times people found me in the middle of attempting. Both times I was in an isolated place; that was God, I know that now. Today, I feel blessed to have almost arrived at the other side of these childhood traumas.

"Now, I am on my way to become a counselor. My long-term goal is to earn a Master's Degree and specialize in working with children and youth. I want to use the gift of compassion for others whot are hurting, especially kids, that I have gained from all the pain I have gone through in my life.

"I started using drugs at 14 years old by smoking weed, then by drinking and doing meth. By the time I was 15, I was an addict. I did drugs because I wanted to fit in with all my so-called friends. I used drugs as a way to escape my problems. I loved the thrill of partying. It gave me a sense of knowing that there was always someone to hang out with me. I got clean at 18, worked, and went to school. Graduated at 19 from high school and went to Community College. I was taking classes to become a district attorney. At 22, I got promoted to shift supervisor at my job; I loved it! I got to be bossy. I am an only child, so being bossy is my specialty. I had a princess attitude and only did drugs because it gave me a social life with people like me.

"I met my son's father at 24, and we fell in "lust" immediately. Shortly after meeting him, we moved in together. I wanted a sense of belonging to someone. I was working, going to school, and paying all the bills. He, on the other hand, lay on the couch playing video games. In my mind that was ok because I was a very dominate person. Within one year, my world had become a living nightmare. I had started using meth again and ended up getting busted on campus for selling drugs. My consequences were that I wouldn't be able to attend that school anymore, and since I was almost done and ready to transfer, I was no longer allowed to continue Administrative of Justice classes. That's about the time my world came crashing down right before my very eyes.

"I had been working at my job as a supervisor for two years. Again, I enjoyed it very much. However, I took advantage of my power and let my addiction get the best of me once again. I remember it like it was yesterday. It was a hot summer day in June as I was setting up our new 4th of July display when I saw the head of loss prevention walk in. Whenever a company head shows up, someone always gets fired! I got paged to the office, and I assumed it was because of all the theft we were having in our store. I walked in and I was asked to have a seat. The company head then told me that the store was investigating some specific activities that had been going on in the store.

"As the the questioning started, I realized that this was about me. I was being investigated for writing bad checks and getting money back on a closed account. (Guilty!) The reason I hadn't been caught sooner was because I was overriding my own checks and forcing them to go through. Needless to say, I was in the office for what felt like ever, and I was charged with fraud.

"I was terminated. Everything I had ever worked hard for in my life was gone. I was left with a car, a dog, and a boyfriend, homeless and scared, not knowing what was coming next.

"The next year was pretty much a blur. All I remember was getting high and living on the streets or off of the Russian River. I became what I hated the most in the world, a junkie! My addiction had started to spiral, and I began slamming dope. I hated my life, and every day I woke up hoping that I would just die. My boyfriend and I fought all the time over stupid things. He would put his hands on me every chance he got, and I would let him, with the hope that each time he would kill me and stop my misery.

"I wasn't feeling all that great and decided to take a pregnancy test. I found out I was pregnant. I tried everything in my power to quit using drugs. Nothing seemed to help. Fast-forward to February 3, 2011: I went in to have my sonogram done and found out at five months that my son was healthy, brain, lungs, and heart all normal. I quit using meth that day. I gave birth to a healthy baby boy. I was then told by the nurses that I had tested positive for Valium and that they were calling Child Protective Services.

"My life forever changed that day; all I wanted was to be a mom, and I felt as if my actions in the past were about to make that impossible. I was interviewed by a CPS worker who made the recommendation that I attend a treatment program and go into a homeless shelter without my son's father. It was the biggest decision I ever had to make, and I chose to be a mother that day. I went to a homeless shelter and enrolled in a drug program that I believed saved my life. I learned how to get back on my feet and started working again.

"My story shows that I had everything, lost everything, and am working slowly to getting it back. I am far from where I wish to be, but my persistence and strength made it possible to be where I am today. I do believe that hitting 'rock bottom' became the solid foundation upon which I rebuilt my life."—Anonymous

Critical Thinking

OVERVIEW: FETAL DRUG ANALYSIS

Refraining from drug and alcohol use is paramount in a child's developmental stages from the womb to adulthood. It is pivotal in a child's life to have parents who understand that drug and alcohol abuse may harm a growing embryo in any form and amount. Misuse can lead to a range of damage from mild to catastrophic to life-threatening deformities causing failures in body systems. Possibilities include drug-induced damage or failure of organs, heart damage, heart failure, brain underdevelopment, brain death, and missing or deformed limbs. Problems in later youth and adult stages of life may not show up for years.

Examples include cocaine, which is known for the effects of low birth weight, smaller head, and smaller frame. Heroin's effects range from mild addiction and withdrawals to death. The drug can cause miscarriages, premature births, or stillbirths. There is also some evidence that suggests heroin use causes behavioral problems and brain underdevelopment. Methamphetamine and amphetamines can cause placental abruption, fetal death due to a lack of oxygen, premature birth, and infant withdrawals. Potential lasting effects include learning difficulties and developmental issues that can arise all throughout life.

Marijuana is often touted as the drug that causes no harm. Scientific evidence and research seems to paint a different picture. THC can affect the brain's ability to learn and its cognitive functions. Researchers have found that babies under the influence of marijuana have a slower response to visual stimuli and verbal communications (crying) that may indicate neurological problems. There is also a higher rate of learning gaps in cognitive thinking, problem solving, and memory. Problems like premature labor or low birth rates and SIDS death can also occur. Research is still being conducted on THC in breast milk and its effects.

What is difficult, if not impossible, to measure is whether adult emotional and behavioral patterns of violence, child abuse, or neglect are a direct result of fetal drug exposure in the womb, along with social and economic factors. A strong indicator is that of learned behavior from the parent by perpetuating addiction and behaviors from generation to generation.

There is really no safe drug. All have the potential for adverse effects on the fetus. The goal is community outreach and educational services for mothers to prevent unhealthy long-term outcomes.

WISH

Medicines Explained:

https://www.youtube.com/watch?v=MHC91r-Zs6A

Receptors Made Simple:

https://youtu.be/HkLoHfvCPCk

Basic Introduction to Drugs, Drug Target, and Drug Interactions:

https://www.youtube.com/watch?v=u49k72rUdyc

Pharmacology Drug Binding:

https://www.youtube.com/watch?v=QZUjBZLLZkM

Introduction to Pharmacokinetics:

https://www.youtube.com/watch?v=mp93nPUzHqM

Pharmacology Mechanism of Action:

https://www.youtube.com/watch?v=FvPLoxsC_LM

Factors Affecting Drug Distribution:

https://www.youtube.com/watch?v=8zYIEiXvSZY

Drug Sandbox

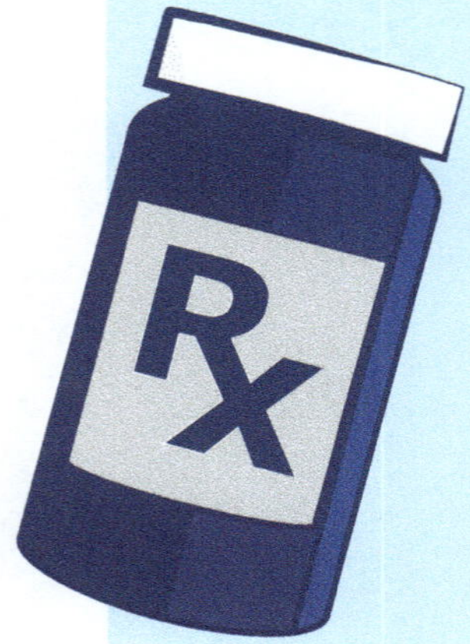

IMPORTANT WORDS TO KNOW!

Agonist
Antagonist
Receptors
Chemical Messengers
Mechanism of Drug Action
Half-life
Therapeutic Effect
Systemic Effect
Therapeutic Range
Prophylaxis
Drug Interaction
Additive Effects
Summation
Synergism
Antagonism
Routes of Administration
Parenteral Administration
Intravenous
Intramuscular
Inhalation
Subcutaneous
Pharmacokinetics
Absorption
Distribution
Metabolism
Elimination
Pharmacodynamics
Local Effect
Systemic Effect
Ceiling Effect
First-pass Effect
Side Effect
MEC, Minimum Effective Concentration
MTC ,Minimum Toxic Concentration
Onset of Action
Therapeutic Window
Duration of Action

Community Connections

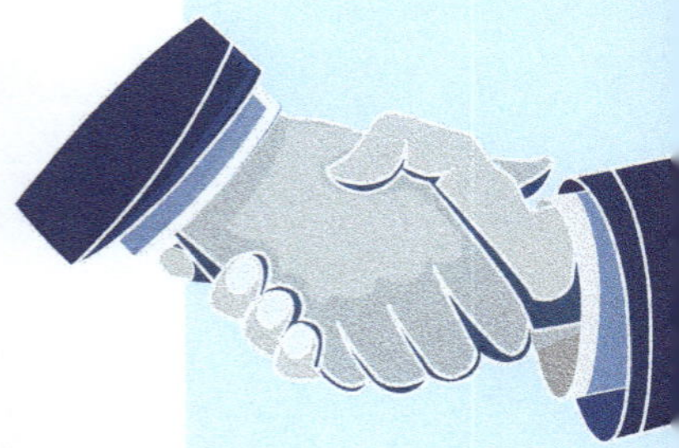

SEEKING SAFETY: A TREATMENT MODALITY

"Seeking Safety" was the first empirically-studied treatment for the dual diagnosis of PTSD/substance abuse" and "has been studied more than any other approach (Implementing Seeking Safety Therapy for PTSD and Substance Abuse). Seeking Safety was originally designed to treat complex trauma clients who suffer from co-occurring conditions and is "based on the principles of prioritizing safety, integrating treatment for both disorders, reinforcing strengths, and instilling hope" (Schmitz 490). The name Seeking Safety expresses its main concept: "When a person has both substance abuse and PTSD, the urgent clinical need is to establish safety." It is set up in a way that both substance abuse and PTSD are addressed at the same time. This seems to be a more cost-effective way for treatment that better meets the client's needs in a sensitive manner and has a higher rate of succeeding (Implementing Seeking Safety Therapy for PTSD and Substance Abuse). "It is used as a general stabilization model to teach coping skills even if a client does not have any history of PTSD or substance use problems" (Treatment Innovations).

Seeking Safety: A Model to Address Trauma and Addiction Together states that:

Most Americans at some point in their lives survive one or more incidents: violence, child abuse, domestic violence, military combat, rape, car accidents, natural disaster (such as a hurricane), life-threatening illness, and industrial incidents. For most people, the impact of trauma fades relatively soon, typically within one to three months. But for others, trauma problems can persist for years and even decades.

In Seeking Safety, a client can start from the beginning of treatment. One does not have to attain stabilization of his or her addiction before beginning treatment.

Implementing Seeking Safety Therapy for PTSD and Substance Abuse states:

If clients have addictive or impulsive behavior in addition to substance abuse (e.g., cutting, binging, gambling), clients are guided to apply the safe coping skills taught in Seeking Safety to those behaviors as well.

The session begins with a check-in of each client. He or she is asked, "What good coping skills have you done since the last session?" Once everyone has checked-in (which is not mandatory), a quotation is read and clients are asked, "What is the main point of the quotation?" Variations in the way these questions are asked are not recommended because it has been proven to work best when sticking with this wording of the questions (Implementing Seeking Safety Therapy for PTSD and Substance Abuse). Actively rehearsing skills through role play, think-aloud, and other varying practices help build the skills that are usable in life. This type of therapy supports the "learn by doing concept" (Schmitz 491). There is a semi-structured format. The sessions are extremely flexible in that they can be done in any order.

The topics are diverse. Clients and clinicians can decide together which topics and handouts should or will be addressed. Each topic is independent of the others. They can be done in any order (Implementing Seeking Safety Therapy for PTSD and Substance Abuse). A benefit of sessions that work in this way is that clients can enter or exit at any time. "Examples of Seeking Safety topics include Honesty, Creating Meaning, Setting Boundaries in Relationships, Taking Good Care of Yourself, Compassion, Coping with Triggers, Healing from Anger, and Recovery Thinking" (Seeking Safety: A Model to Address Trauma and Addiction Together).

The length of treatment can vary among clients. Some clients may only have time for a few sessions if they are in inpatient treatment, but others who are in a long-term residential treatment facility will have more time to cover the topics. They may be able to go over topics two or three times. There is also an open door policy. Clients can leave and come back at any time. This policy is similar to AA and NA groups. Clients need not master the skills or topics; they are offered a variety of coping skills to choose from and pick what works best for them (Implementing Seeking Safety Therapy for PTSD and Substance Abuse). Another benefit of this treatment modality is it can be facilitated by staff without advanced degrees. This is beneficial because most staff members do not have advanced degrees. "It does not appear to exceed the training, licensure, or ethical limits of substance abuse counselors." If it does go beyond their scope of knowledge and education, they may refer out for more specialized treatment (Implementing Seeking Safety Therapy for PTSD and Substance Abuse).

Seeking Safety is an evidence-based model of therapy (Seeking Safety: A Model to Address Trauma and Addiction Together). If not followed as it is intended, it could result in negative effects. Therefore, these guidelines should be followed. Too much talking by the clinician can make it seem like school rather than therapy. The rule "80/20" is suggested; the clinician talks 20% of the time to the client's 80% of the time. Second, the wording of questions should not be changed from the format. Research has proven the wording to be very important, and straying from this can have a different effect. Third, the tone of the group is important. In many other groups, confrontation may be supported. Lastly, single-gender groups support the comfort of the client. If sessions were to be co-ed, many clients may not feel comfortable in sharing trauma which is sexual or physical in nature (Implementing Seeking Safety Therapy for PTSD and Substance Abuse).

Trauma and substance abuse often go hand-in-hand. People may turn to substances to cope with their trauma. Addiction and substance abuse can also lead to trauma. This can range from driving while intoxicated to more serious crimes such as sexual violence (Seeking Safety: A Model to Address Trauma and Addiction Together). Through Seeking Safety, clients may see for the first time the link between PTSD and SUD (substance abuse disorder) which can relieve the feelings of shame and guilt that are attached to each disorder individually. Exploring how the two may be linked, how one may trigger the other, and how they came about in relation to each other can help to establish safe coping skills for both (Schmitz 492). The goal is always to help clients grow, love who they are, and love who they can become.

The difference between Seeking Safety and other therapy modalities is that Seeking Safety stays in the present. It teaches clients a broad range of coping skills that they may never have learned growing up or may have lost along the way as their addiction progressed. All of the coping skills apply to both trauma and addiction. Providing this kind of treatment can help motivate the client to see the connection between his or her trauma and addiction.

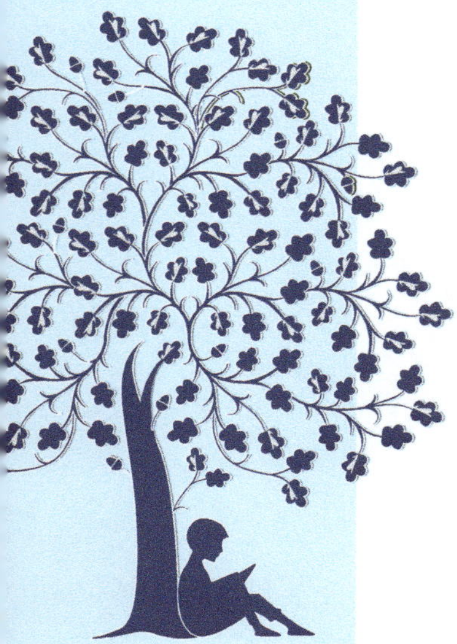

End Of Chapter Review Questions

Select the letter that matches the following words with their appropriate meanings:

1. Half-life	a. Preventive effect of a drug
2. Therapeutic effect	b. Elimination of 50% of drug in circulation
3. Systemic effect	c. Desired action of a drug in the treatment of a disease or symptom
4. Therapeutic range	d. Optimum dosage scope for effectiveness with the least toxicity
5. Prophylaxis	e. Generalized, all-inclusive drug effect on the body
6. Pharmacodynamics	f. The study of drugs

7. Pharmacokinetics — g. The study of harmful effects of drugs on living tissue
8. Toxicology — h. Controlled substances assigned by their medical usefulness and potential for abuse
9. Pharmacology — i. The study of the action of drugs on living tissue
10. Drug schedules — j. The study of drug absorption, distribution, metabolism and excretion

Indicate if the following statements are true (A) or false (B):

11. OTC means the drug is over-the-counter and available for purchase without a prescription.

12. Once a patent expires, the drug may be produced in the generic form with a considerable lower price differential.

Multiple Choices: Select the best answer from the choices given:

13. Which of the following definitions best describes pharmacokinetics?
    a. The absorption, distribution, metabolism, elimination of drugs in the body over a period of time
    b. The absorption and elimination of drugs by the body over a period of time
    c. The distribution of drugs through the body over a period of time
    d. The elimination of drugs from the body over a period of time

14. What is a drug interaction?
    a. Allergy to a drug
    b. Fatal reaction to a drug
    c. Tolerance to a drug
    d. Combined effect of two drugs

15. Reasons for different routes of administration include:
    a. Convenience
    b. Desire a rapid onset
    c. Target and deliver the drug to the site of action
    d. Prolong the duration of action
    e. All of the above are correct

16. Ciclopirox (Penlac) is an antifungal used to treat onychomycosis, a type of nail fungus. The directions say to apply the lacquer to each nail daily. What type of effect will the ciclopirox have?
    a. Local effect
    b. Systemic effect
    c. Ceiling effect
    d. First-pass effect
    e. Side effect

17. Parenteral administration includes all of the following, except:
    a. Intravenous
    b. Intramuscular
    c. Inhalation
    d. Subcutaneous

18. A newspaper ad is recruiting healthy adults, ages 18–45 years, for a clinical drug trial. The drug is named Rememberal for the treatment of Alzheimer's. Recruits are to take the drug orally and to come in once a week for labs and an examination. The drug has a ____________ effect.
    a. Local
    b. Systemic
    c. Ceiling
    d. First pass
    e. Side

19. Sources of drugs include:
    a. Plants and animals
    b. Minerals and synthetics
    c. Bioengineering
    d. All of the above

20. Ethical reasons for medication use include all of the following except:
    a. Disease prevention
    b. To cure disease
    c. To control the disease process

d. Palliation
e. Recreational abuse

21. Synergism can be defined as:
    a. The combined effect of two drugs
    b. The combined effect is more than the sum of their individual effects
    c. One drug cancels another drug's effect
    d. One drug enhances another drug's effect

22. Decreased drug effect after chronic administration is known as:
    a. Incompatibility
    b. Antagonism
    c. Additive effects
    d. Synergism
    e. Tolerance

23. When the combined effect of two drugs is less than the sum of their individual effects, it is called:
    a. Synergism
    b. Antagonism
    c. Additive effects
    d. Summation
    e. Tolerance

24. When the combined effect of two drugs is greater than the sum of their individual effects, it is called:
    a. Synergism
    b. Antagonism
    c. Additive effects
    d. Summation
    e. Tolerance

25. When the combined effect of two drugs, each producing the same biologic response by the same mechanism of action, is equal to the sum of their individual effects, it is called:
    a. Synergism
    b. Antagonism
    c. Additive effects
    d. Summation
    e. Tolerance

Applications: Assessment of Usage and Relevance

1. Describe the various routes of drug administration. What are the advantages and disadvantages of each method?
2. How do drug half-lives relate to the effectiveness of a dose of a drug?
3. Label the components of a typical dose-response curve.
4. Describe how drug action is terminated and drugs are eliminated from the body.
5. Explain the different types of drug action and drug interactions.

KEY

1. B	8. B	15. E	22. E
2. C	9. A	16. A	23. B
3. E	10. C	17. C	24. A
4. D	11. A	18. B	25. C
5. A	12. A	19. D	
6. D	13. A	20. E	
7. E	14. D	21. B	

REFERENCES

Portrayal Paradigm

Marriage and Divorce Patterns by gender, race, and educational attainment. Bureau of Labor and Statistics. n.p., 2013. Web. 14 Sept. 2015. http://www.bls.gov/opub/mlr/2013/article/ marriage-and-divorce-patterns-by-gender-race-and-educational-attainment.ht.

"The Science of Drug Abuse and Addiction." NIH, National Institute on Drugs Abuse, n.p., n.d. Web. 14 Sept. 2015. http://www.drugabuse.gov/publications/reserch-reports.

"Illegal Drugs in Pregnancy." Baby center. n.p., 2015. Web. 14 Sept. 2015. http://www.babycentre.co.uk/a541318/illegal-drugs-in-pregnancy.

Mannino, Davis J., ed. Introduction to Human Sexuality. Guernewood Park: Teddybear Publishing, 2005.

Community Connections

"Implementing Seeking Safety Therapy for PTSD and Substance Abuse." Web. Sept. 2015.

Schmitz, Martha. "The Case: Treating Jared Through Seeking Safety." Journal Of Clinical Psychology 69.5 (2013): 490–493. MEDLINE with Full Text. Web. 2 Sept. 2015.

"Seeking Safety: A Model to Address Trauma and Addiction Together." Web. 8 Sept. 2015.

CHAPTER THREE

THE BRAIN

Chapter Objectives

1. Discern the importance of neurotransmission.
2. Define the primary neurotransmitters and their function on behavior, mood, and physiology.
3. Differentiate the pharmaceutical agents that affect neurotransmitters.
4. Characterize the neural synapse.
5. Identify instances to optimize patient management.

Positive Affirmations

> "Regret is much larger than the task."
>
> —Gail Beale

Pharmacology

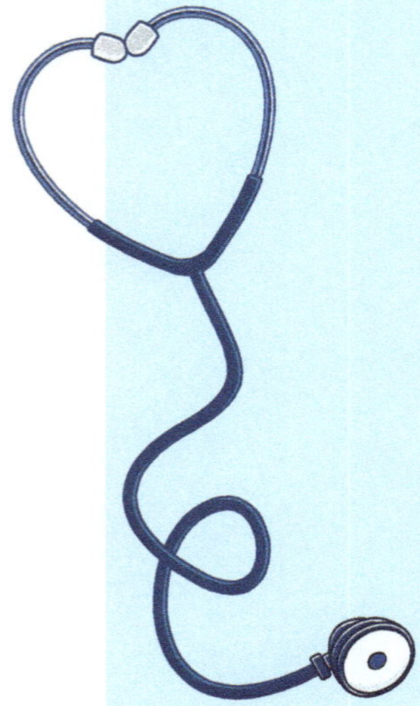

NEUROTRANSMITTERS

Neurotransmitters Overview Watch: https://www.youtube.com/watch?v=ThsT8HOeOtQ

Pharmacology is concerned with the study of drug action and biological receptors. Neurotransmitters are brain chemicals that communicate information throughout the brain and body. The brain uses neurotransmitters to communicate, such as telling the heart to beat, the lungs to breathe, and the stomach to digest. They can affect mood, sleep, concentration, weight, and cause unhealthy symptoms when out of balance. Neurotransmitter levels can be decreased by stress, poor diet, drugs, alcohol, and caffeine.

Since the discovery by Austrian scientist Otto Lowie of a chemical he called "Vagusstoff" in 1921 (now known as acetylcholine), scientists have identified some 100 different molecules that meet the criteria for being regarded as neurotransmitters, and their exact numbers are still unknown. Simply stated, a neurotransmitter is a messenger of neurologic information from one cell to another. These messengers are serotonin (5-HT), gamma-aminobutyric acid (GABA), dopamine (DA), norepinephrine (NE), epinephrine (Epi), acetylcholine (Ach), glutamate (Glu), and endorphin.

There are two different kinds of neurotransmitters, inhibitory and excitatory, which have different signaling effects in the brain. Excitatory neurotransmitters (dopamine, norepinephrine, epinephrine, and glutamate) stimulate the brain. They excite the neighboring neuron, increasing the activity. Inhibitory neurotransmitters (GABA and serotonin) calm the brain, balance mood, and are easily drained when the excitatory neurotransmitters are overly active. They inhibit the neighboring neuron, dampening or suppressing the activity.

A neurotransmitter must:

- Be manufactured in the neuron
- Be released by a nerve impulse (action potential) from the presynaptic terminal
- Hit the postsynaptic receptor and cause an effect
- Be inactivated, metabolized, or removed from the receptor by a process

- **Inactivation** can occur via reuptake, the process of the body reabsorbing the neurotransmitter back into the neuron.
- **Metabolism** occurs by destruction of the neurotransmitter by body enzymes in enzymatic degradation.
- **Removal** occurs when the neurotransmitter and receptor separate from each other. The neurotransmitter drifts or diffuses out of the synaptic cleft.

Molecules of neurotransmitters are stored in small packages called vesicles (Figure 3.1). Neurotransmitters transmit signals across a chemical synapse from one neuron (nerve cell) to a target neuron, muscle cell, or gland cell. They are released from synaptic vesicles and diffuse into the synaptic cleft, where they bind to specific receptors on other synapses. Communication of information is accomplished by this movement of electrical and chemical means which causes an effect.

The four major neurotransmitter imbalances include, "everything we do, such as all our movements, thoughts, and feelings, are because of the chemical or electrical signals. Neurons communicate with each other through neurotransmitters, which interact with receptors located throughout the

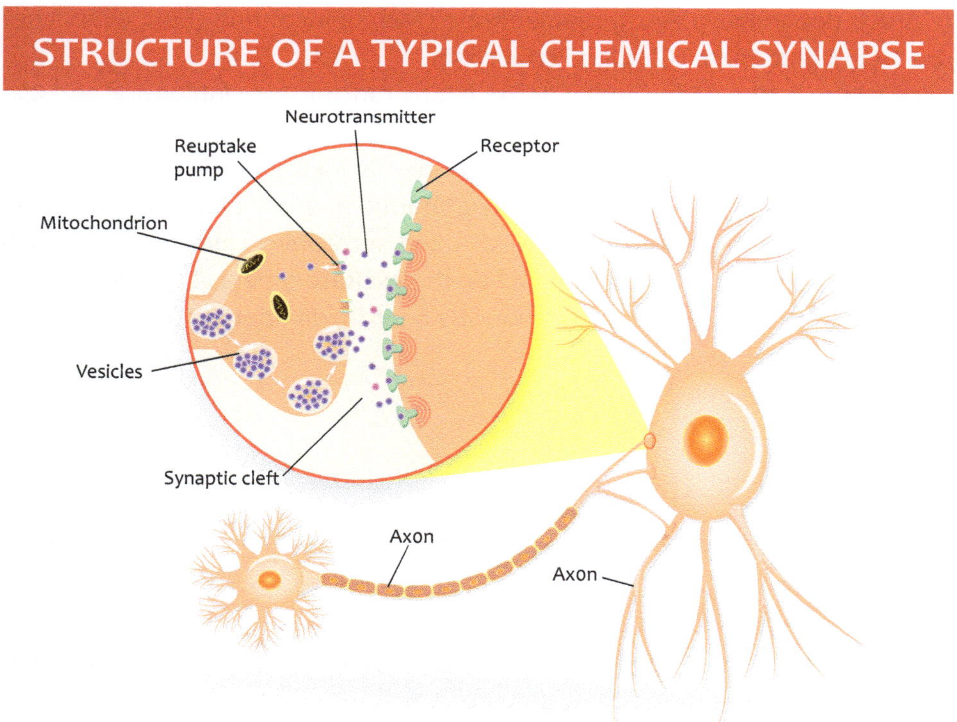

Figure 3.1 Copyright © Depositphotos/edesignua.

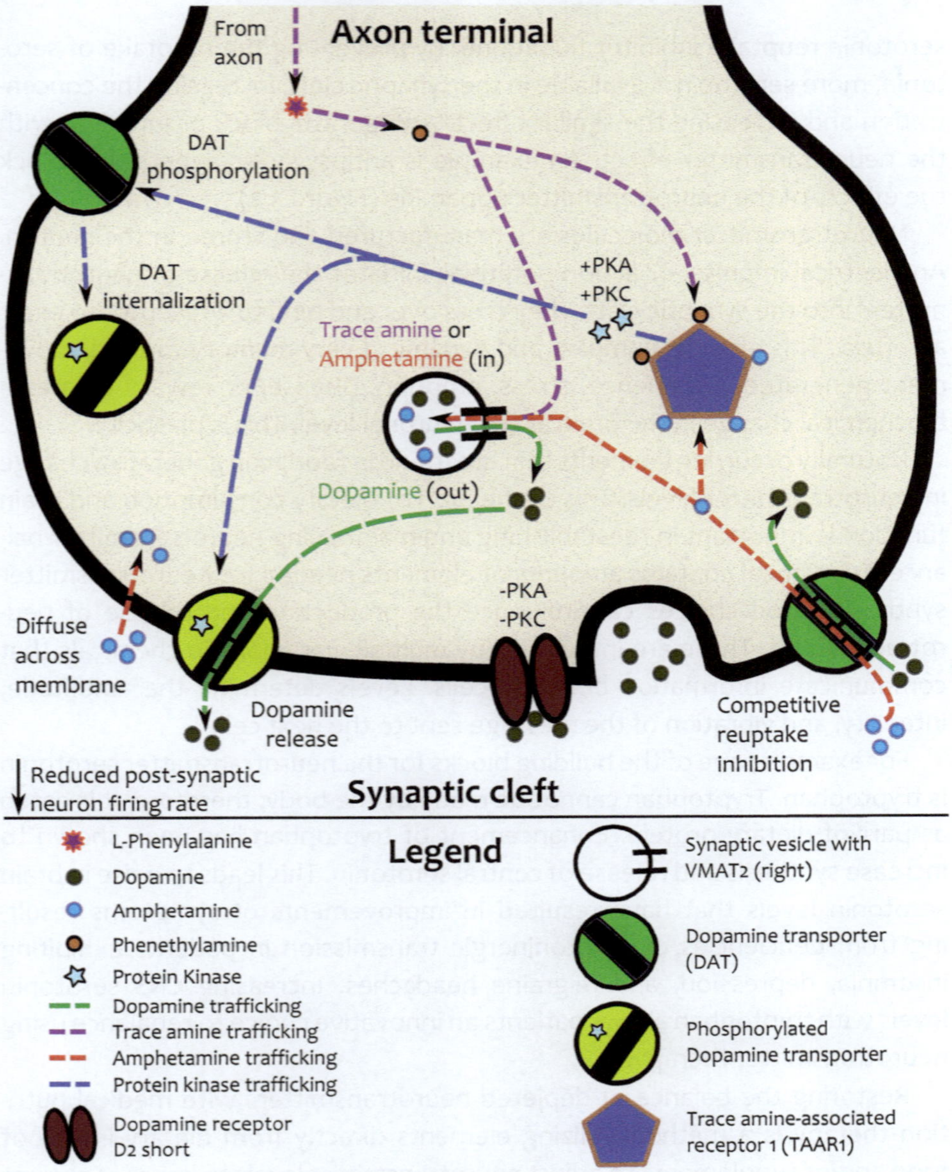

Figure 3.2 Copyright © Seppi333 (CC BY-SA 3.0) at https://commons.wikimedia.org/wiki/File:TAAR1_Dopamine.svg.

brain and body to regulate a wide variety of processes, including emotions, fear, pleasure, joy, anger, mood, memory, cognition, attention, concentration, alertness, energy, appetite, cravings, sleep, and the perception of pain. Neurotransmitters affect every cell in the body."

Substances that affect neurotransmitters are agonists and antagonists. Their effect can be as an agonist (similar) or antagonist (blocker). Agonists simulate or assist the effect of the neurotransmitter. An example is the serotonin reuptake inhibitor fluoxetine. By preventing the reuptake of serotonin, more serotonin is available in the synaptic cleft, increasing the concentration and increasing the similar effect. Antagonists block or interfere with the neurotransmitter effect. An example is antipsychotic agents that block the effects of the neurotransmitter dopamine (Figure 3.2).

Neurotransmitter molecules are manufactured and stored in the neuron. An electrical impulse, or action potential, initiates the release of neurotransmitters into the synaptic cleft. They cross over and bind to a receptor to exert an effect. This effect is complex and dynamic. Every memory formed, movement generated, experience, stress, emotion, disease, or reward creates a biochemical change in the brain at the neuronal level. This is plasticity.

Naturally occurring elements that are found in foods can generate a change in neurotransmitter levels. This connection of dietary consumption and brain function is important in reestablishing and maintaining neurotransmitter balance. Every meal contains amounts of elements needed for neurotransmitter synthesis. Food choices can influence the production and release of neurotransmitters. These are influenced by multiple variations in chemicals that communicate information between cells. Levels determine the amplitude, intensity, and vibration of the message sent to the next cell.

For example, one of the building blocks for the neurotransmitter serotonin is tryptophan. Tryptophan cannot be made by the body; therefore, it is eaten as part of dietary protein. Enhancement of tryptophan has been shown to increase synthesis and release of central serotonin. This leads to a rise in brain serotonin levels that have resulted in improvements of symptoms resulting from deficiencies of serotoninergic transmission in patients exhibiting insomnia, depression, and migraine headaches. Increasing CNS serotonin levels with tryptophan allows patients an innovative choice to rebalance using neurotransmitter therapy.

Restoring the balance of depleted neurotransmitters with medical nutrition therapy is a method utilizing elements directly from dietary intake of food and/or supplements to adjust neurotransmitter levels to improve patient outcomes, thinking, feeling, and behaving. Prescription medication therapy is a method utilizing pharmaceutical compounds to exert an effect.

FUNDAMENTAL NEUROTRANSMITTERS

Gamma-aminobutyric acid (GABA) is an inhibitory neurotransmitter that is sometimes called "Nature's Valium." GABA regulates the brain's excitability.

It is the lead neurotransmitter in seizure prevention and in the management of epilepsy. GABA acts like a brake on the excitatory neurotransmitter system. It promotes a calming effect, eases anxiety, and enhances sleep. When GABA is too high or too low, it can be caused by an excitatory neurotransmitter, like glutamate, that is going off too often in the brain. GABA will be released to balance the over-stimulating excitatory. The inhibitory effects of GABA can be increased by sedative-hypnotic agents, such as benzodiazepines and barbiturates. Alcohol is a commonly used and abused sedative-hypnotic whose effects on GABA contribute to the antianxiety and sedative properties of alcohol.

Low levels of GABA have been connected to:

- Insomnia
- Depression
- Anxiety

GABA supplements are not effective in producing a calming, sleep effect because they are unable to cross the blood brain barrier. Prescription antidepressants and sleeping medications are able to cross this brain barrier and stimulate the body's existing GABA receptor sites.

Fermented foods such as kimchi (fermented cabbage) are the only dietary source of GABA. Other lactobacillus-fermented foods containing GABA include kefir, miso, sauerkraut, tempeh, yogurt, and Pu-Erh Tea. Flavonoid-rich foods (phytonutrients found in plant-based foods) may enhance GABA function. They include berries, citrus fruits, apples, pears, tea, cocoa, and wine. Medicinal plants include chamomile flowers, feverfew, linden flowers, and passionflower.

GABA-driven personalities have the tendency to share the common attributes of stability, consistency, sociability, and concern for others. They are nature's most dependable people. They can be counted on to show up at work every day and be there when others need them. At work, GABA-dominant people are the ones who set goals, organize projects, schedule activities, and keep others on task. Their punctuality, objectivity, practicality, and confidence make them excellent employees. Organization is paramount to them—at work, at home, and in their social life. They're the ones in the group who stay focused on the matter at hand. They are the consummate team player both metaphorically and literally.

Serotonin (5-HT) 5-hydroxytryptamine (5-HTP) is an inhibitory neurotransmitter; it does not stimulate the brain. The appropriate balance of serotonin affects pleasure, mood, body temperature, appetite, and advances peacefulness and contentment to balance any excessive excitatory neurotransmitter. Changes in serotonin levels and uptake sites are associated with affective disorders like depression. Stimulant medications, caffeine, and nicotine can cause serotonin levels to decrease over time. Serotonin also regulates other things, such as carbohydrate cravings, sleep cycle, pain control, and appropriate digestion. Low serotonin levels are connected with decreased immune system function.

Serotonin is a precursor of melatonin, the hormone that is released by the absence of light and aids in sleep. Tryptophan is an amino acid building block of serotonin, which is a component of milk. Tryptophan-rich foods include turkey, chicken, lamb, beef, liver, halibut, shrimp, salmon, snapper, scallops, spinach, kelp, seaweed, spirulina, peas, beans, and mushrooms. Essential fatty acids increase serotonin production. They include omega-3 fatty acids (fish, walnut, flax oil), omega-6 fatty acids (canola, grapeseed, safflower, sunflower, wheat germ oils), and gamma-linoleic acid (spirulina or blue-green algae, black currant, evening primrose, borage oils).

Symptoms and conditions of serotonin imbalance include:

- Loss of pleasure and enjoyment;
- Anxiety;
- Bipolar disorder;
- Insomnia;
- Migraines;
- Irritable Bowel syndrome;
- Obsessive Compulsive disorder;
- Fibromyalgia;
- Depression;
- Indigestion;
- And many others.

The amino acids and co-factors required for serotonin production and utilization include:

- Vitamin B6 in the form of Pyridoxal-5-Phosphate; it is an essential cofactor in the production of serotonin but can be depleted by overconsumption of alcohol;
- Vitamin B 12 in the form of methylcobalamin;
- Folic acid;
- Magnesium;
- Niacinamide; and
- Iron deficiency experienced with anemia.

Serotonin-driven personalities know how to live in the moment. Realistic and impulsive, they are highly responsive to sensory input. They're active participants in life who thrive on change. They take their vacations at a different spot each year. They try new foods, new hobbies, and new friends, and they have a natural disdain for order, structure, and authority. They're optimistic, cheerful, easygoing, and the life of the party. A serotonin-dominant person gravitates to trades or professions that offer a variety of tasks, an ever-changing environment, and interactions with different people. In relationships, they can be romantic and passionate, but they also love their independence and often refuse to be tied down.

Dopamine (DA) is a neurotransmitter that is both excitatory and inhibitory. It is associated with the pain, pleasure, and reward centers—our body's natural amphetamine. Dopamine facilitates metabolism, energy, alertness, focus, happiness, relaxation, motivation, and eases depression and pain. It assists in establishing desires and goals and triggers our reward center. Body functions, including increased heart rate, blood pressure, digestion, motor coordination, cognition, mood, attention and learning, are regulated by dopamine. Dopamine is one of many substances that keep our brains lubricated and functioning. When this delicate balance is in harmony, the brain sends the proper signals.

In appropriate amounts, this reward-system neurotransmitter will keep us feeling good. Stimulant medications for ADD/ADHD, nicotine, caffeine, and illicit abuse substances can push dopamine into synapse and temporarily improve focus. A negative consequence in overstimulating dopamine too much and for too long is a permanent decrease of dopamine later in life. Dopamine in excessive levels can cause behavior changes and enhance personality traits, ranging from anxiety to schizophrenia, so much so that daily existence becomes a fractured reflection of what it once was. These underlying traits exist. They are always there. It is now that the expression of these traits is dramatically amplified.

The reduction of dopamine to low levels affects movement and motor areas of the brain, resulting in difficulties of movement like Parkinson's disease. Enhanced dopamine production comes from foods rich in phenylalanine and tyrosine: chocolate, beef, pork, fish, turkey, eggs, cheese, blueberries, spirulina, chicken, yogurt, milk, almonds, peanuts, tofu, and most soy-based products.

An imbalance of dopamine may produce symptoms or conditions of:

- Parkinson's disease
- Depression
- Fatigue
- Social anxiety
- Heavy menstrual cycles
- High or low blood pressure
- Loss of libido
- Learning disorders
- ADHD
- Addictions
- Schizophrenia
- Hopelessness
- Low stress tolerance

The amino acids and cofactors required for dopamine production and utilization include:

- Mucuna pruriens and its components, including L-Dopa, which is converted into dopamine in the brain.
- Beta-Phenylethylamine (PEA) influences endorphins attributed to feeling pleasure, improving attention, and relieving depression. Chocolate is a rich source of PEA.
- Blueberry extract contains a rich and potent source of antioxidants proven effective in free-radical quenching of dopamine-rich neurons of the central nervous system.
- D, L-Phenylalanine (DLPA) is an essential amino acid precursor to dopamine. It is effective in managing depression, moods, and reducing pain perception. N-Acetyl-Tyrosine is another amino acid that is a precursor of dopamine.

- Glutathione cofactors include selenium, lipoic acid, and n-acetyl-cysteine. They are essential nutrients for the synthesis of glutathione that help protect the neuronal tissue responsible for dopamine production.
- Vitamin B6
- Folic acid and B12 (deficiencies can result due to hypothyroidism, use of oral contraceptives and estrogen replacement, antacid use, decreased levels of hydrochloric acid, and h pylori infections).

Dopamine driven personalities are not new. They are likely to be strong-willed individuals who know what they want and how to get it. They are highly rational, more comfortable with facts and figures than feelings and emotions. They can be self-critical but do not accept criticism or negative feedback from others. These people function well under stress, focusing intently on the task at hand. They are tireless and typically need less sleep than average. Strategic thinking, invention, and problem-solving are the hallmarks of these individuals. In their personal lives, they like activities related to knowledge and intellect. They tend to establish personal relationships easily but may have trouble nurturing them. As highly rational people, they have trouble understanding that many people believe feelings are more important than reason.

Acetylcholine (Ach) is a multifaceted receptor substance; nicotinic and muscarinic receptors are found in the nervous system. Nicotinic receptors are so called because they respond to nicotine agonists, such as the alkaloid of the tobacco plant. They are located on muscle cells and certain neurons in the brain. Stimulation produces effects on performance, mood, vigilance, memory, concentration, focus, muscle coordination, cardiovascular function, and pain perception. Ach is responsible for REM (dream) sleep. There appears to be a link between low acetylcholine and Alzheimer's disease as a 90% loss of acetylcholine is seen in the brains of people suffering from Alzheimer's.

Acetylcholine is not found in food. It is synthesized from choline, which is found in lecithin and phosphatidyl choline. These elements are in eggs (yolks contain lecithin), milk (source of choline), organ meats (beef liver contains choline), brussel sprouts, broccoli (sources of choline), peanuts, and whole wheat products.

Acetylcholine-driven personalities are quick thinkers, highly creative, and open to new ideas. Flexibility, creativity, and impulsivity open them up to trying almost anything as long as it offers the promise of excitement and something new; they are not afraid of failure. They love to travel and have a quest for lifelong learning. These people also tend to be extremely sociable, even charismatic. They love making new friends and put a lot of energy into all of their relationships, whether at work, at home, or in the community. They are eternally optimistic and, thus, "they are quite popular with a broad range of people.

Epinephrine (adrenalin) is the excitatory neurotransmitter that is secreted from the adrenal glands on the kidneys in response of stress (physical, mental, emotional) as perceived from fear or injury. Epinephrine increases heart rate, blood pressure, bronchodilation, metabolic rate, blood glucose concentration, and it places the body in the fight-or-flight mode. It is increased when ADHD-like symptoms are present. Long-term insomnia and stress can cause epinephrine levels to decrease.

Norepinephrine (noradrenaline) is an excitatory neurotransmitter that is connected to stimulating the body. Norepinephrine makes epinephrine (adrenalin), as well. It places our bodies in fight-or-flight mode to a perceived threat. It increases our heart rate, blood pressure, and triggers the sympathetic nervous system. At high levels, norepinephrine can cause anxiety, insomnia, and a shift in mood. Low levels of norepinephrine can cause decreased focus, low energy, and sleep-cycle problems.

Glutamate has an excitatory effect and is important for fast excitatory signaling in the part of the nervous system involved in behavioral and physiological functions. It is the most commonly found neurotransmitter in the central nervous system. This complex neural network includes learning, plasticity, memory, cell death in some disorders, and potentially the development of psychopathologies, including addiction and schizophrenia. Excessive glutamate levels may result is cell death. Amyotrophic lateral sclerosis, ALS (aka Lou Gehrig's disease), results from excessive glutamate production. Glutamate depletion may occur from infection, surgery, or trauma. Since the body synthesizes glutamate, supplementation may not be necessary. Rich glutamate sources are fish, beef, chicken, pork, turkey, beans, milk, yogurt, ricotta cheese, cottage cheese, raw spinach, cabbage, and parsley.

Endorphin is short for endogenous morphine and is our bodies' pain medication similar to the opioids. As an inhibitor, it is involved in pain reduction and pleasure. Endorphin is the neurotransmitter that allows bears and other animals to hibernate.

CAR IMAGE METAPHOR

- GABA is "the braking system."
- Serotonin is "the battery."
- Dopamine is "the gas in the car."
- Acetylcholine is "the accelerator."

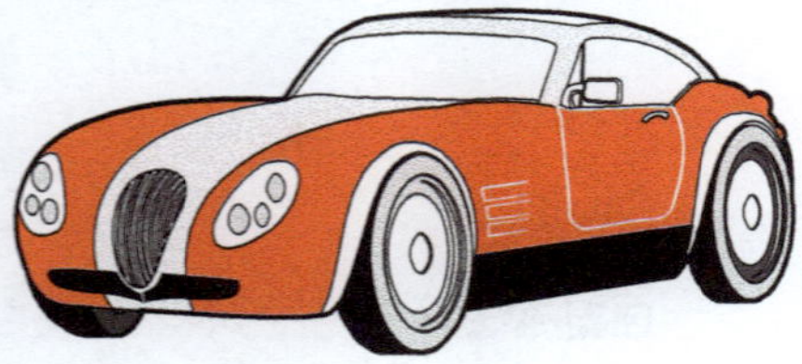

Figure 3.3 photothailand, "Sports Car," https://openclipart.org/detail/93385/sport-car. Copyright in the Public Domain.

Reframe the main neurotransmitters as a car! This picture adds depth to developing an understanding of the brain and how it works. Conceptually seeing neurotransmitters like serotonin as a battery gives insight into how energy stores are used to face the world. The braking (or calming effect) of GABA through Medical Nutrition Therapy is a tool. We have all experienced the gas and accelerator effects of dopamine and acetylcholine. This framework helps to build an understanding of brain chemistry in a more holistic fashion—the whole is truly greater than the sum of the parts.

It is important to keep neurotransmitters balanced for our mental, emotional, and physical health. Sometimes a chemical imbalance can be improved simply by getting regular exercise, eating a proper diet with omega-3, making sure you are taking in enough vitamin D, placing yourself in healthy environments, keeping the level of stress down, as well as utilizing coping skills, acupuncture, and talk therapy with a doctor or therapist. Different types of medication can also be helpful.

Supplemental information: If you have any interest regarding the correlation of neurotransmitters and personality visit http://www.spwb.com/articles/brainarticle.html. This comprehensive website is succinct, with reference to a book for more in-depth knowledge. The website points out that "medical advances of today and the very near future—gene therapies, nanotechnology, targeted monoclonal antibodies, cloning, and more—will allow us to repair or replace damaged and diseased bodies' parts and raise the average life expectancy to 100 years or more. The problem with this advancement is that the studies suggest that 40% of those reaching 85 and nearly 100% of those reaching 120 will be senile. Of what use is living to a ripe old age if we cannot enjoy it or even be aware that we're alive?

CONTROL OF BODY FUNCTIONS—NERVOUS SYSTEM

Physiology of the Nervous System:

https://www.youtube.com/watch?v=hzXVe4RS8-A

Autonomic Nervous System (ANS)—An overview of anatomy, divisions, receptors, and neurotransmitters:

https://youtu.be/Y_5J7NG85CY

Sympathetic Nervous System:

https://www.youtube.com/watch?v=oIDgBlCHVsA

Autonomic Nervous System

- Unconscious activation to maintain life:
- Respiration, pupils, heartbeat ...

Somatic Nervous System

- Conscious purposeful activation:
- Posture, muscles, locomotion ....

Sympathetic (Adrenergic) Autonomic Nervous System (SANS)

- Fight, flight, faint, freeze, fawn
- Increase heart rate
- Increase contractility
- Bronchodilate
- Renin release

Selected Receptor Sites of the SANS System

Alpha Receptors

- Alpha 1
- Alpha 2

Beta Receptors

- Beta 1
- Beta 2

Norepinephrine

Epinephrine

Parasympathetic (Cholinergic) Autonomic Nervous System

- Relax, conserve, rest, digest
- Reduction in heart rate
- Reduction in contractility

Selected Receptor Sites of the PANS System

- Acetylcholine
- Nicotinic sites
- Muscarinic sites

Alpha Omega

"My name is Sophie; I am a grateful recovering addict. I went to the party early and stayed late. My experiments with mind- and mood-altering substances began with nicotine when I was 11. The experiments became habit and then addiction. I have been in recovery for seven and one-half years now. I got clean at 55. I was able to be in one of the first groups to take the Hep C wonder drug, Sofusbrivir. I was cured within the 12-week treatment. My dark passenger that I carried with me since 1975 was finally gone. I returned to school last fall.

"My substance misuse took me to some of the darkest places that experience can, including being homeless in the Tenderloin district of San Francisco. I have come to believe that the trauma and desperation that resulted from my plummeting into addiction is a true blessing of my life. Now, I live each day in gratitude with the intention of being of service. My family and I are rebuilding our relationships. They are stronger, more intimate, and vital than before. Recovery has also given me the gifts of faith, hope, and true friendships. It has nurtured my loving and caring side. Where I once thought, 'what's in it for me?' I now think, 'it's not all about me.' I no longer see it as I deserve but that I am open to receive.

"It is said that ongoing recovery work is like peeling an onion; I see it more as the cycle of a flower blooming. Recovery has given me the strength, perspective, and esteem to walk through what I ran from all my life. I embrace the work I do to continue the cycle of my flower blooming. I accept what will wither and fall away and have faith for what will bud and bloom. This process I am describing has changed and continues to change my brain. I think differently because I have acted differently. (I love neuroscience!) I have a life I never allowed myself to dream of. Gratefully, I tell you my story is not over, but just beginning. "—Anonymous

Critical Thinking

PICKING THE OPTIONS THAT GIVE US THE MOST OPTIONS

"It wasn't very long ago that my options were very limited. I had pigeonholed myself into taking a very narrow road with no forks. The option that I picked led to years, actually decades, of addiction to hardcore drugs, chronic criminal behavior, toxic relationships with the exact same type of woman over and over again, an apathetic antisocial perspective of the world, low self-esteem that was fueled by no self-respect, and an existence consisting of loneliness, rage, self-centeredness, desperation, and misery. Obviously, I had picked the wrong option. How exactly did I go from living like that to having the rich, fulfilling life that I have today?

"There are many ways to answer that question. I believe that it comes down to making the choice to stop picking the option that gives me the fewest options. The process involved me admitting to myself that I was not doing a good job at making choices. It involved me surrendering the only way of life that I had ever known and having faith that there had to be a better way to live. I couldn't get more out life with the same thinking and the same doing as I always had. In recovery, we have an acronym, H.O.W., Honesty, Open-mindedness, and Willingness, and I believe that these three principles are the options that give me the most options. If I practice these principles, I have a whole world full of options in front of me. If I don't, I can go right back to the only option that I had before.

"I must say that there is freedom that comes with having options. I get to pick the kind of person that I want to be every morning. I set my goals as high or as low as I want. I can be productive or lazy. There are the more tangible options: Do I want to be a therapist, counselor, social worker, or something else? Do I want to squat or bench press today? Which major should I go with in school? Should I marry my girlfriend or should we keep our relationship off the books? These are far better options than I had a couple years ago."—Anonymous

WISH

Neural Synapse:

https://www.youtube.com/watch?v=LT3VKAr4roo

Neurons and What They Do:

https://www.youtube.com/watch?v=vyNkAuX29OU

Brain and Neurotransmitters:

https://www.youtube.com/watch?v=6uMcdpiV094

Brain Pleasure Centers:

http://thebrain.mcgill.ca/flash/a/a_03/a_03_cr/a_03_cr_que/a_03_cr_que.html

Pleasure Centers Affected by Drugs:

http://thebrain.mcgill.ca/flash/a/a_03/a_03_cr/a_03_cr_par/a_03_cr_par.html

Brain Mechanisms of Pleasure and Addiction:

https://www.youtube.com/watch?v=de_b7k9kQp0

Avoiding Pain:

http://thebrain.mcgill.ca/flash/a/a_03/a_03_cr/a_03_cr_dou/a_03_cr_dou.html

How Addiction Changes your Brain:

https://www.youtube.com/watch?v=5f1nmqiHIIl

The Addicted Brain:

https://www.youtube.com/watch?v=Ap1yAFL_HdI

GABA and Glutamate:

https://www.youtube.com/watch?v=_q6tBL9iWvM

Serotonin, Dopamine, and your Brain:

https://youtu.be/sr9ol6r91cA

Serotonin and Tryptophan:

https://www.youtube.com/watch?v=8bPVWRPWhEU

Dopamine:

https://www.youtube.com/watch?v=Nt5AkMDLIdo

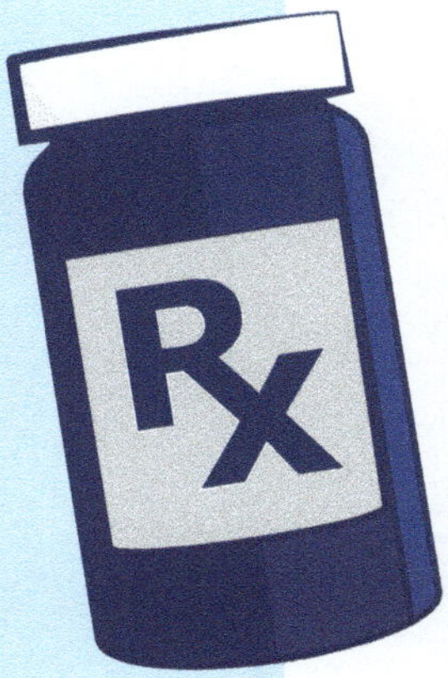

Drug Sandbox

IMPORTANT WORDS TO KNOW!

Neurotransmitters
Excitatory Neurotransmitters
Inhibitory Neurotransmitters
Neuron
Synapse
Reuptake
Enzymatic Degradation
Neurotransmitter Drift or Diffusion
Synaptic Cleft
Agonists
Antagonists
Receptor Sites Interaction
Plasticity
Neurotransmitter Therapy
Medical Nutrition Therapy
Prescription Medication Therapy
GABA
5-HT
DA
Ach
Epinephrine (Adrenalin)
Norepinephrine (Noradrenaline)
Glutamate
Endorphin
Autonomic Nervous System
Somatic Nervous System
Sympathetic (Adrenergic) Autonomic Nervous System (SANS)
Selected Receptor Sites of the SANS System
Parasympathetic (Cholinergic) Autonomic Nervous System
Selected Receptor Sites of the PANS System

Community Connections

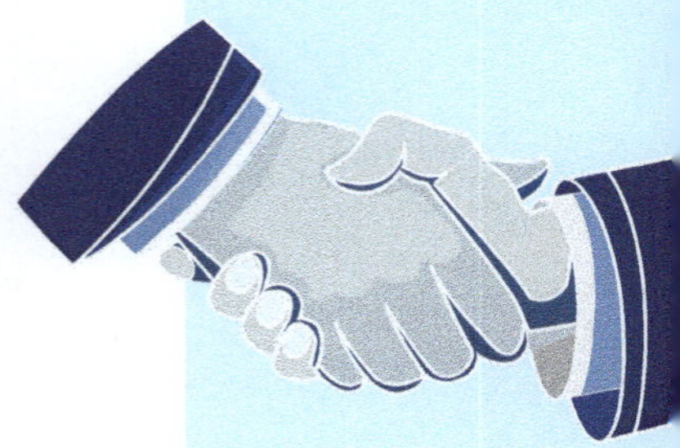

Throughout human history, drug use and spirituality have been intertwined and perceptually contradictory, depending on the particular branch of spiritual belief and the nature of the substance. In Christianity and Judaism, wine plays an integral part of central rituals, and in Native American religions, psychoactive drugs are an element of spiritual awakening. In others, the mirror inverse is seen. Islam and Mormonism ban intoxicating beverages and drug use. The prohibition against drug or alcohol use is seen in many branches of mainstream Christianity, as well, and older members of American society may still remember taking a "temperance pledge" at their own churches as youths. This intersection of substance use or prohibition is curious.

One line of thinking postulates that substance use and spirituality may be tied together by the natural processes in the human body that lead to or cause specific euphoric experiences. For example, research has been conducted which ties the euphoric feelings produced by some types of music to the release of endogenous opioids (Miller and Bogenschutz, 2007). The feelings of euphoria that some people experience in specific spiritual or religious ceremonies is not unlike the feelings produced by particular drugs, such as opioids. In addition, the out-of-body, seemingly transcendent experience that can be produced by some psychoactive agents is considered by some to be an element of the divine and integral to the expanded perspective that some associate with spirituality.

In opposition to these viewpoints is a perception essentially of modern idolatry; drug addiction displaces any other interests or priorities, leaving the addict with a model of the world that places obtaining and using drugs as the priority. (Miller and Bogenschutz, 2007). When external factors are the central motivators for existence, a person's focus, by definition, is the worldly and not the spiritual. Many involved in modern treatment programs consider spirituality and drug use to be entirely at odds; where one exists, the other cannot. Whether or not this is a rational assessment is fairly subjective though there is an extensive body of research exploring the topic of addiction, recovery, and spiritual belief.

Within the constructs of spirituality and religion, a common theme among those new to 12-Step Programs is the need to differentiate between spiritual belief and the religious. Many who seek these programs have a bias against organized religion or have simply chosen to not be practitioners. In order to address this issue, the authors of Alcoholics Anonymous chose to use alternative terms for God, placing emphasis on the ability to personally choose an individual conception of a power greater than oneself. The impact of this choice is extremely significant. Many who are not willing to associate themselves with a particular religious group or to establish a concrete notion of divine power are, therefore, still able to conceptualize in the abstract an individualized higher power, and, thus, establish personal spiritual practices (R. Walker et al, 2013, p. 1234).

Religion is commonly defined as a social construction particular to a certain community or culture which has particular prescribed practices and belief systems. In organized religion, the emphasis is on conforming to the established belief system, not establishing ones' own. Spirituality, however, can be, but is not necessarily, linked to any religious affiliation. According to Katsogianni and Kleftaras (2015), spirituality is most concerned with ones' personal relationships to larger, transcendent realities, such as God or the universe. Spirituality is an aspect of an individual and can be expressed both positively and negatively.

Positive expressions on spirituality might include a belief that life fundamentally has meaning, that the world and individual lives serve a positive purpose, and that the universe is an ordered, intentional place. These examples are one component of spirituality's ability to make personal connections and define beliefs in whatever way appeals to the individual. Conversely, negative spirituality may be expressed in feelings of meaninglessness, insecurity, depression, or overt aggression (Katsogianni and Kleftaras, 2015). That individual, who does not believe in the connection of life forms to each other or in the collective meaning of the universe as a whole, exists in what has been described as an existential vacuum (Frankl, 1969). The result of this kind of thinking has been shown in research to be linked to poor mental health, increased incidence of suicide or suicidal gestures, and significantly increased abuse of substances. (Katsogianni and Kleftaras, 2015).

An inverse relationship exists between spirituality and addiction showing that levels of positive spirituality and depressive thinking were negatively correlated while negative spiritual outlook and depressive thinking were positively correlated. To restate those results, the more positive spirituality a person possessed, the less likely he or she was to be depressed. Additionally, the same study established that depression and drug abuse were positively correlated. When those findings are looked at as a collective whole, the result is that there is empirical evidence that positive spirituality and drug abuse are inversely related. A person who has strong spiritual belief is less likely to be addicted to a substance.

A metric for the expression of addiction in spiritual terms was established in four component parts by Galanter (2007). They are as follows:

- Loss of sense of purpose in life due to substance use.
- Feeling of inadequate social support because of addiction.
- Moral qualms about substance use in spite of persistent use.
- Loss of the will to resist temptation when the substance is available.

These components are one attempt to establish a concrete measure for identifying the intersection of spirituality and addiction. However, one shortfall of this metric is implied causation. In the study conducted by Katsogianni and Kleftaras, there was an attempt made to show correlation but not necessarily an overt expression of causation. Implicit in the above components outlined by Galanter is the assumption that drug use is causing these negative spiritual outcomes. Without that assumption, one might conceive that lack of positive spirituality may be the precursor to drug abuse and not the final outcome. The following is another attempt at constructing criteria for the self-reporting of spiritual belief (Sussman, et al, 2013, p. 1205):

- People might simply be asked how spiritual they are or whether they hold spiritual beliefs (Sussman, Nezami, and Mishra, 1997).
- Another type of item assesses a person's participation in spiritual groups or events (Berry, 2005; Sussman et al., 2005).
- A third type of spirituality item assesses a person's engagement in spiritual experiences, such as meditation and prayer or trying to obtain solace from a higher power (Carroll, 1993; Kass et al., 1991; Sussman, Nezami, and Mishra, 1997).
- A fourth type of spirituality item taps subjective self-beliefs, such as a sense of purpose, feeling peaceful, feeling a sense of harmony, sense of forgiveness, or sense of connectedness (Koenig, 2008; Underwood and Teresi, 2002).

When this type of metric is used, there is a basis for establishing spiritual belief without implicitly stating that the lack is caused by drug use. One of the issues concerning the study of spirituality and addiction is the issue of defining spirituality. If spiritual belief is, by definition, individualistic, then how should it be measured and by what criteria? Research has been conducted using various measures of spirituality, but the factor that remains consistent is that spirituality can essentially only be measured through self-reporting. The individual is the only one qualified to establish whether his or her rate of spirituality is low or high and increasing or decreasing across a span of time.

Consistent with this approach is research by Conner, et al (2008). Participants were asked to self-report specific aspects of religious and spiritual belief and were grouped as: consistently highly religious/spiritual, consistently low, increasing (across a 12-month period), and decreasing (across the same period). The outcome was that those in the consistently high and increasing groups showed significantly fewer days of drug use than those in the other two groups. Results also indicated that these differences were dependent on spiritual group attendance and maintenance of spiritual practices but not on religious group attendance or religious practices.

Spirituality is an ongoing tool. The findings in Conner, et al (2008) lead to the conclusion that in order to create or maintain lower levels of drug use or addictive behaviors, an individual must establish and maintain not only positive spiritual beliefs but also corresponding practices. The example of this in addiction treatment is 12-Step Programs. AA and NA both emphasize the essential nature of spiritual awakening and experience in order to effect change in addiction patterns. There is controversy around 12-Step Programs and their alliterations. Whether or not 12-Step Programs are the best or the only method of creating and maintaining spiritual practices and group attendance is debatable. All aspects of spirituality have a voice that calls to the individual. The individual has choice and discernment. It is given that each person's path will lead him or her to certain information, beliefs, conclusions, and methods of practice. What is a necessity is establishing and maintaining some kind of positive spiritual life in the process of addition recovery.

End Of Chapter Review Questions

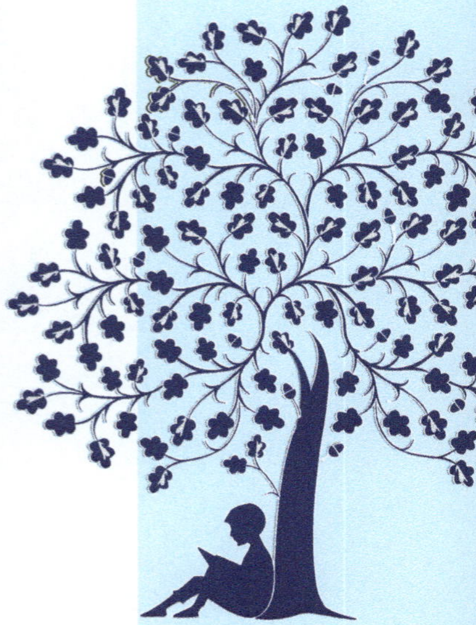

Matching: Using the list below, select the best answer:

1. The excitatory neurotransmitter that is secreted from the adrenal glands on the kidneys in response of stress.
2. The neurotransmitter that is both excitatory and inhibitory. It is associated with the pain, pleasure, and reward centers; it is our body's natural amphetamine.
3. The inhibitory neurotransmitter; it does not stimulate the brain. The appropriate balance affects pleasure, mood, and advances peacefulness and contentment.
4. The endogenous morphine and our bodies' pain medication.
5. The inhibitory neurotransmitter that is sometimes called "Nature's Valium."
6. It is the most commonly found neurotransmitter in the central nervous system and is important for fast excitatory signaling in the parts of the nervous system involved in behavioral and physiological functions.
7. The multifaceted receptor substance; nicotinic and muscarinic receptors in the nervous system.
8. The excitatory neurotransmitter that is connected to stimulating the body into fight-or-flight mode to a perceived threat.

a. GABA
b. 5-HT
c. DA
d. Ach
e. Epinephrine (adrenalin)
f. Norepinephrine (noradrenaline)
g. Glutamate
h. Endorphin

Indicate if the following statements are true (A) or false (B):

9. Antagonists interfere with neurotransmitter function.

10. Agonists simulate neurotransmitter function.

11. Neurotransmitter function is a balance of excitatory and inhibitory effects.

12. The presence of neurotransmitters allows the brain to communicate information.

13. Neurotransmitters are mostly made up of amino acids.

Multiple Choices: Select the best answer from the choices given:

14. Neurotransmitters include:
    a. Dopamine
    b. Norepinephrine
    c. Serotonin
    d. All of the above

15. Heart rate increases when beta-1 receptors are stimulated. A patient takes a drug that binds on the beta-receptors and he or she experiences an increase in heart rate. This drug was a:
    a. Beta antagonist
    b. Beta agonist
    c. Beta inhibitory
    d. Beta blocker

16. The major excitatory transmitter in the brain is:
    a. Glutamate
    b. Ach
    c. Dopamine
    d. AMPA

17. The major inhibitory transmitter in the brain is:
    a. GABA
    b. Glycine
    c. Glutamate
    d. Norepinephrine
    e. Serotonin

18. The peripheral side effects of the psychostimulants resemble activation of:
    a. The SANS
    b. The PANS
    c. The central nervous system
    d. The parasympathetic nervous system
    e. The skeletal nervous system

19. Ach, DA, NE, GABA, and 5-HT are examples of:
    a. Phases of the sleep cycle
    b. Substances of abuse
    c. Primary motor and thought CNS neurotransmitters
    d. Classifications of panic disorders
    e. None of the above

20. The psychostimulants are thought to act most importantly through which neurotransmitter?
    a. Dopamine
    b. Acetylcholine
    c. Histamine
    d. Norepinephrine
    e. None of the above

Applications: Assessment of Usage and Relevance

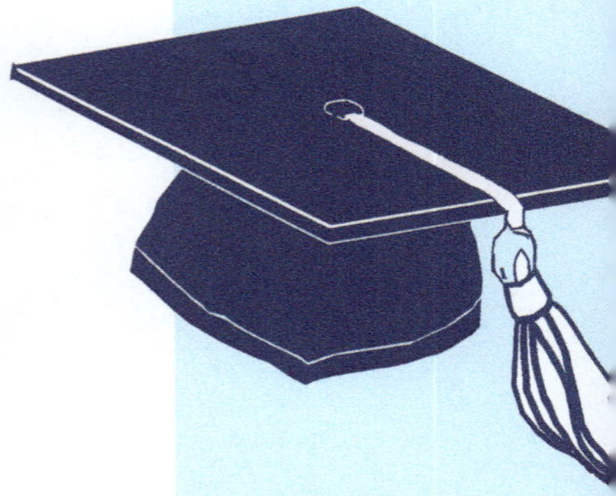

1. Explain the ways that a drug may act to affect synaptic transmission (agonist, antagonist, partial, etc.).

2. What is dopamine? What does it do? What is a dopamine receptor? What occurs in a dopamine deficient and excessive state?

3. What is acetylcholine? What does it do? What is an acetylcholine receptor? What occurs in an acetylcholine deficient and excessive state?

4. What is GABA? What does it do? What is a GABA receptor? What occurs in a GABA deficient and excessive state?

5. What is serotonin? What does it do? What is a serotonin receptor? What occurs in a serotonin deficient and excessive state?

6. Describe the pharmacodynamics of ethyl alcohol, including all affected neurotransmitter systems covered so far.

KEY

1. E	6. G	11. A	16. A
2. C	7. D	12. A	17. A
3. B	8. F	13. A	18. A
4. H	9. A	14. D	19. C
5. A	10. A	15. B	20. A

REFERENCES

Fundamental Neurotransmitters

Golan, D. E., Tashjian, A. H, Armstrong, E. J., and Armstrong A. W. (2012). Principles of Pharmacology The Pathophysiologic Basis of Drug Therapy (3rd ed.). Philadelphia, PA: Lippincott Williams & Wilkins.

Murphy, J. E. (2012). Clinical Pharmacokinetics (5th ed.). Bethesda, MD: American Society of Health System Pharmacists.

Stahl, S. M. (2013). Stahl's Essential Psychopharmacology Neuroscientific Basis and Practical Applications (4th ed.). New York, NY: Cambridge University Press.

Growdon, J. H., Wurtman, R. J.: Contemporary Nutrition: Nutrients and Neurotransmitters. New York State J. Med., Sept. 1980.

Chara, Paul J., Jr. "Neurotransmitters." Salem Press Encyclopedia of Health. n.p.: Salem, 2014. N. pag. Ers. Web. 13 Dec. 2015.

"Neurotransmitters." Causes, Effects, Drug, People, Used, Brain, Personality, Mood. n.p., n.d. Web. 14 Dec. 2015.

"Neurotransmitters." The Four Major and the Neurotransmitter Imbalances. n.p., n.d. Web. 14 Dec. 2015.
http://www.spwb.com/articles/brainarticle.html.
www.neurogistics.com.
https://faculty.washington.edu/chudler/chnt1.html.
webspace.ship.edu/cgboer/genpsyneurotransmitters.html.
http://health.howstuffworks.com/mental-health/anxiety/nutritional-therapy-for-anxiety-and-depression.htm.
http://www.bbwca.com/neurotransmitters/neurotransmitters-therapy/.
http://www.livestrong.com/article/478780-a-list-of-foods-with-the-highest-gaba/.
http://www.livestrong.com/article/288554-list-of-foods-with-serotonin/.
http://www.livestrong.com/article/249869-dopamine-rich-foods/.
http://www.livestrong.com/article/392875-food-sources-of-acetylcholine/.
http://www.livestrong.com/article/249890-list-of-foods-that-contain-glutamine/.

Community Connections

Conner, B. T., Anglin, M. D., Annon, J., and Longshore, D. (2009). Effect of Religiosity and Spirituality on Drug Treatment Outcomes. Journal Of Behavioral Health Services & Research, 36(2), 189–198. doi:10.1007/s11414-008-9145-z.

Katsogianni, I. V., and Kleftaras, G. (2015). Spirituality, Meaning in Life, and Depressive Symptomatology in Drug Addiction. International Journal Of Religion & Spirituality In Society, 6(2), 11–24.

Longshore, D., Anglin, M. D., and Conner, B. T. (2009). Are Religiosity and Spirituality Useful Constructs in Drug Treatment Research? Journal Of Behavioral Health Services & Research, 36(2), 177–188. doi:10.1007/s11414-008-9152-0.

Miller, W. R., and Bogenschutz, M. P. (2007). Spirituality and Addiction. Southern Medical Journal, 100(4), 433–436.

Sussman, S., Milam, J., Arpawong, T. E., Tsai, J., Black, D. S., and Wills, T. A. (2013). Spirituality in Addictions Treatment: Wisdom to Know...What It Is. Substance Use & Misuse, 48(12), 1203–1217. doi:10.3109/10826084.2013.800343.

Treloar, H. R., Dubreuil, M. E., and Miranda, R., Jr. (2014). Spirituality and Treatment of Addictive Disorders. Rhode Island Medical Journal, 97(3), 36–38.

Walker, R., Godlaski, T. M., and Staton-Tindall, M. (2013). Spirituality, Drugs, and Alcohol: A Philosophical Analysis. Substance Use & Misuse, 48(12), 1233–1245. doi: 10.3109/10826084.2013.799020

CHAPTER FOUR

STIMULANTS

Chapter Objectives

1. Recognize descriptions of ephedrine, cocaine, amphetamines, methamphetamine, nicotine, and caffeine.
2. Describe the scope of each of their mechanisms of action.
3. Explain addiction treatment modalities both pharmacologic and non-pharmacologic for each.
4. List methods of smoking cessation therapies.
5. List symptoms of caffeinism and caffeine withdrawal.

Positive Affirmations

"There is more to life than increasing its speed."

—Gandhi

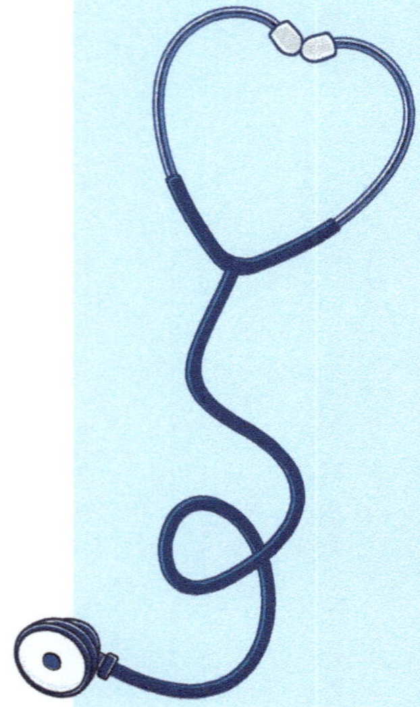

EPHEDRINE

Ephedrine is a stimulant derived from the Chinese plant ma huang. The drug has been used for thousands of years to treat a multitude of ailments ranging from aching bones and joints to breathing problems, asthma, weight loss, colds, and flu. Presently, it is available for symptomatic relief of asthma attacks, shortness of breath, chest tightness, as well as a bronchodilator and decongestant. It can be found over-the-counter as an herbal stimulant commonly used for flu symptoms or asthma. Ephedrine sulfate stimulates the cerebral cortex and has a potent effect on the central nervous system. This sympathomimetic drug directly and indirectly stimulates alpha and beta receptors. It is an agonist at noradrenaline receptor sites and has the ability to increase the release of serotonin and dopamine. As a stimulant, ephedrine activates **thermogenesis** in the body. This effect results in speeding up the heart rate, causing the metabolism to expedite. It is due to this increased metabolism that ephedrine is used as a weight-loss supplement.

Pseudoephedrine, a **decongestant**, relieves symptoms by reducing swelling and congestion by constricting blood vessels in the nasal passages and widening the lung airways for easier breathing. It is used for relief of shortness of breath, chest tightness, and wheezing due to bronchial asthma. Ephedrine is also marketed as an **appetite suppressant** for weight loss and as a **concentration booster**; its natural form comes from the plant Ephedra equisetina.

Ephedrine's chemical structure is similar to **methamphetamine.** It has the potential to be abused as it can be synthesized into the illegal substance. Ephedrine is available for consumers to purchase at a local pharmacy although sales of it are highly monitored. Retailers cannot sell more than three packages or nine grams in a single transaction and may not sell the drug to anyone under the age of 18. Ephedrine's well-established presence in the over-the-counter (OTC) drug market has made it extremely difficult to ban it completely. In 1997, the FDA proposed an attempt to regulate the amount of ephedra (from which the herb ephedrine is derived) by limiting a dose to 8 mg, with no more than 24 mg per day. The attempt failed due to lack of evidence showing that low dosages of ephedrine are unsafe, that the agent is mixed with a multitude of other herbals and medications that would result in a huge recall, and that potentially many companies would close down, resulting in thousands of lost jobs.

Common side effects of ephedrine are similar to those produced by **amphetamines**: anxiety, dizziness, insomnia, tremor, nervousness and restlessness, tension, spinning sensation (vertigo), headache, nausea, and loss of appetite (anorexia), palpitations, sweating, confusion, delirium, convulsions, and hallucinations. Potential side effects of **pseudoephedrine** include fast, pounding, or uneven heartbeat; severe dizziness; dangerously high blood pressure; and unusual weakness. Extreme cases can even cause vomiting, hallucinations, and severe mental disorders. It also increases blood pressure, which, in turn, speeds up the metabolism of ephedrine takers.

Misuse has resulted in severe liver damage. Serious and sometimes deadly drug interactions occur when ephedrine is mixed with other stimulants. Cardiovascular side effects associated with large doses of ephedrine have included tachycardia and palpitation. Precordial pain and arrhythmias have been reported following administration of ephedrine injection. Hypertension, stroke, and myocardial infarction have also been reported. Ephedrine poisoning may show up as fever, chills, vomiting, tachycardia, and hypertension. The most dangerous symptoms are the high blood pressure and rapid or irregular heartbeat that can lead to death.

Commonly used as a stimulant to focus concentration and suppress appetite, dosage is dependent upon the route of administration, indication for use, and patient-specific factors. Ephedrine is available in injectable and oral forms. The oral dosages of pseudoephedrine for an adult vary depending on the dosage form. Immediate release is 30 to 60 milligrams every four to six hours, sustained release is 120 milligrams every twelve hours, and a sustained release suspension is 45 to 100 milligrams every twelve hours. All are taken as needed and are not to exceed 240 milligrams per day. The sustained release suspension would provide less than the maximum daily dosage if taking the highest recommended dosage of 100 milligrams twice a day while the immediate release and sustained release forms would meet but not exceed the maximum amount of 240 milligrams. Initial dose: 25 to 50 mg orally every three to four hours. Maximum dose: 150 mg per day in divided doses. Parenteral: Initial dose: 25 to 50 mg IM or subcutaneously every three to four hours or 5 to 25 mg slow IV push (over at least 15 minutes); may be repeated in five to ten minutes, if necessary. Maximum dose: 150 mg per day in divided doses.

Cocaine

Coca leaves are used indigenously in South America, and cocaine was isolated from coca in 1859 by Albert Niemann. Cocaine addiction insidiously gains financial, psychological, and physical control over the user. It is the second most common emergency department visit (number one is alcohol in combination with other drugs) (DAWN 2004). Street names include snow, coke, blow, toot, white lady, crack, ready rock, and rock candy. It has the capability of being smoked, sniffed, swallowed, or injected. Cocaine is classified as a central nervous system stimulant and a schedule CII drug. It is incredibly addictive in nature and also has the potential to be very dangerous, resulting in brain damage, weight loss, and death.

Cocaine addiction primarily affects dopamine. This is the neurotransmitter responsible for rewards in the brain. Levels of dopamine increase, which cause the euphoria commonly associated with the drug. It also has a similar effect on norepinephrine, which is an additive to the energetic effect of the drug. Enzyme metabolism of cocaine is accomplished by **butyrylcholinesterase (BChE).** This enzyme is found in plasma and in red blood cells. It metabolizes cocaine, aspirin, amitriptyline, and it activates heroin. Red blood cell BChE activity is most effective at metabolizing cocaine. Women have more red blood cell BChE; to varying degrees women are less susceptible to cocaine effects than men. BChE has protectant effects against cocaine toxicity and nerve agent toxicity.

Cocaine Administration

- Powder; most often inhaled (snorted)
- Injected (IV)
- Swallowed (orally or by chewing coca leaves)
- Smoked (freebase)

Pharmacokinetics of Cocaine

- Absorption
  - Intranasal: 20–30%; plasma peaks in 30–60 min
  - Smoked: 6–32%; plasma peaks at 5 min
  - Intravenous: 100%; immediate; 60 sec to brain
- Distribution
  - Easy, quick access to brain
  - Concentration in brain exceeds plasma level
  - Crosses placental barrier freely (crack babies)

Cocaine is rapidly metabolized by the liver. The approximate elimination half-life for oral (50 minutes), nasal (80 minutes), and IV (60 minutes) is short, thus, causing the addict to use the drug every 1/2 hour or less to maintain the high. The cocaine metabolite **enzoylecgonine** appears and lasts 48 hours to two weeks. When alcohol and cocaine are in the body at the same time, this creates the metabolite **cocaethylene**. Cocaethylene acts like cocaine and is more toxic.

Pharmacodynamics of Cocaine

- Acts as a local anesthetic and vasoconstrictor.
- Blocks reuptake of monoamine neurotransmitters.
- Blocking reuptake of dopamine produces stimulation, behavioral reinforcement, and activates the reward center.
- Brain areas of high cocaine activity: ventral tegmental area (VTA); dopamine neurons project to medial prefrontal cortex, nucleus accumbens, amygdala, and hippocampus.
- Cocaine blocks dopamine transporter proteins, increasing the concentration of dopamine.

Signs and Symptoms of Acute Cocaine Intoxication

- Increased temperature, blood pressure, heart rate
- Euphoria, giddiness, boastfulness for 30 minutes, then 60–90 minutes of mild euphoria and anxiety
- Anorexia
- Agitation, insomnia
- Hallucinations
- Seizures, death
- Restlessness, anxiety persists for hours; depression rebound
- Nasal passage damage
- Lung damage
- Intense, short-term high followed by dysphoria
- Death from overdose

Hazards of Use

- Intense psychological and physical dependence
- Life-threatening cardiac dysrhythmias, hypertension, hemorrhagic cerebrovascular accident

High Dose Effects and Safety Risks

- Chronic users
  - Toxic paranoid psychosis
  - Skin eruptions
- Cocaine bugs
- Circulatory collapse
  - Strokes and myocardial infarction
- Psychiatric disorders
  - Psychosis, suicide, delirium

Reinforcement Potential of Cocaine

- Low doses are reinforcing
- Cocaine craving follows
- Self-administration of cocaine persists in the face of punishment
- Withdrawal increases craving
- May heighten sexual interest but does not improve potential or performance

Cocaine exposure in the early months of pregnancy can cause early labor or miscarriage. Cocaine decreases the amount of nutrients and oxygen that are passed to the fetus. Babies known to be exposed to cocaine while in the womb are six times more likely to be born underweight. This carries a 20 times higher risk of being more likely to die in the first month. Those who survive the first month of life are at higher risk of lifelong disabilities, including mental retardation, cerebral palsy, visual and hearing impairment. Cocaine plays a role in **placental abruption** where the placenta is pulled away from the wall of the uterus before labor. This may result in extensive bleeding that can be fatal to both the mother and the unborn baby. After birth, the baby can be cocaine-dependent and suffer from withdrawal symptoms such as tremors, sleeplessness, muscle spasms, and feeding difficulties.

Fetal Effects of Cocaine

- Birth defects include underweight babies, premature babies, and still-born births
- Cardiovascular: heart attacks, respiratory failures, strokes and seizures.
- Cerebral (brain) reduced cognitive performance, information processing, and lack of multitask ability
- Struggles with social interactions, social skills in early childhood, ability to socialize with peers, and the ability to process information in order to be able to respond to situations

- Vasoconstriction of uterus and placenta
  - Stillbirth and preterm labor
- Congenital malformations
  - Aberrant brain and heart development
  - Cerebral infarction and hemorrhage
  - Sudden infant death syndrome (SIDS)
- Neonatal complications
  - Acute fetal withdrawal
  - Neurobehavioral delays
- Educational difficulties, easily frustrated
- Difficulty dealing with stimulation
- Attachment disorder, AD/HD

Presently, there are no proven or FDA-approved medications to treat cocaine addiction. Treatment models begin with a needs analysis to diagnose comorbid disorders, cocaine-related disorders, appropriateness of beginning of abstinence, maintainence of abstinence while treating disorders, and prevention of relapse in particular interrelated multifaceted layers.

Abstinence Pattern Analysis

Crash: Nine hours to four days, "out of it"
Withdrawal: One to ten weeks, craving and relapse
Extinction: Indefinite, cued craving

Pharmacotherapy is varied. **Diazepam, haloperidol**, and **propranolol** appeared to have a **cocaine antagonizing** or **blocking** effect on behavioral symptoms of cocaine. Diazepam, at all doses, provided significant protection against cocaine- and methamphetamine-induced seizures. Propranolol altered the incidence of methamphetamine-induced seizures. Significant protection against cocaine-induced death was afforded by diazepam and propranolol. Significant protection against amphetamine-induced death was provided by haloperidol and propranolol. No agent reduced the incidence of methamphetamine-induced death. The failure of the antagonists to protect against methamphetamine-induced toxicity and death suggested that different mechanisms of toxicity may exist between these drugs. **Dopamine agonists, bupropion or imipramine,** are used in the reduction of cocaine-induced cravings. Future research is pending on **dopamine antagonists.**

The alcohol abstinence treatment, **disulfiram (Antabuse)**, has produced the most consistent reductions in cocaine abuse. Disulfiram causes the alcohol to be indigestible so a person will have a severely unpleasant reaction if combined with alcohol. For utilization in cocaine treatment, disulfiram appears to cause the blockage of a specific form of dopamine. It has been shown to inhibit this chemical, which is an essential component in the production of norepinephrine; thus, making it a double-pronged attack on the effects of cocaine.

When combined with cocaine, the suppression of norepinephrine production combines with a hyperstimulation (which is related to the drug's impact on dopamine), which is extremely unpleasant for the user. However, this is only a theory at present, and it looks like disulfiram may be more of a stepping stone onto more effective treatments for cocaine addiction. The mechanism of action for cocaine inhibition is unclear at this writing.

Research has shown that about 50 percent of patients who abuse heroin in addition to cocaine will benefit from the combination of **buprenorphine and disulfiram** as treatments. Since buprenorphine is already used for the treatment of heroin addiction, this combination of drugs has genuine potential for polysubstance abusers. **Nepicastat,** an inhibitor of dopamine beta-hydroxylase and an enzyme that catalyzes the conversion of dopamine to norepinephrine, is in research phase studies. This agent focuses on the specific neurotransmitter with a reduction in side effects. In combination with buprenorphine, it could be even more effective.

Low-dose sedation with a **benzodiazepine,** like **Valium** or **Xanax**, will assist in dampening the stimulant effect of acute cocaine use. **Antidepressants** are utilized for comorbid difficulties.

Several medications marketed for other diseases (e.g., **vigabatrin, modafinil**, **tiagabine**, **disulfiram**, and **topiramate**) show promise and have been reported to reduce cocaine use in controlled clinical trials. A **cocaine vaccine** that prevents entry of cocaine into the brain holds promise for reducing the risk of relapse.

Behavioral treatments for cocaine addiction have proven to be effective in both residential and outpatient settings. Forms of therapy showing positive results are contingency management, motivational incentives (MI), cognitive-behavioral therapy (CBT), therapeutic communities (TCs) or residential programs, and community-based recovery groups—such as Cocaine Anonymous—that use a 12-Step Program.

Amphetamines and Methamphetamine

Amphetamine's therapeutic classification is similar to natural catecholamine neurotransmitters, epinephrine, norepinephrine, and dopamine. It acts as an **indirect catecholamine agonist**. It blocks norepinephrine reuptake in the presynaptic nerve endings. Symptoms of amphetamine use may be indistinguishable from cocaine use. Street amphetamines nicknames include speed, amp, jelly, rippers, uppers, bennies; dextroamphetamine go by dexies; and methamphetamine tags include crystal, meth, speed, chalk, and black beauties. The pharmacokinetics of amphetamines is in its administration; it is either swallowed in a pill or capsule or injected into veins, the drug causing an orgasmic feeling or rush. Some people create the circumstances of alkalizing the urine to increase the duration of effect. The half-life of the drug is 5–6 hours in a urine pH of 5. The duration of effect jumps to 20 hours if the pH of the urine is 7.

Selected amphetamines have a prescribed use in managing the symptoms of **attention deficit disorder (ADD), attention deficit hyperactivity disorder (ADHD)**, and treatment-resistant depression. Sample diagnostic criteria include inattention, underperforming, failing to notice details, not seeming to listen, easily distracted, lacking follow through and organization, avoiding sustained mental effort and focus, losing things, and being forgetful. Behaviors that include the hyperactivity-impulsivity set include fidgeting, inability to sit still, leaving seat often, running, climbing excessively, difficulty in quiet time, talking excessively, and being characterized as "on the go" and "driven by a motor." Stimulant treatment of ADD and ADHD slows growth in children, which rebounds with abstinence or a drug holiday. About half of the cases persist into adulthood. ADD and ADHD increase the risk of antisocial personality disorder by ten times and quintuple incidence of drug abuse. For a self-test visit: http://www.fmsnutrition.com/adhd_self_testing_or_test.htm.

Pharmacodynamics of Amphetamines

- Peripheral NS effects: **Sympathomimetic**
  - Constriction of blood vessels: elevation of blood pressure, heart rate
  - Irritability, nervousness, mood swings
- CNS effects: **Psychostimulant**
  - Increase in motor activity
  - Insomnia, loss of appetite
  - Hallucinations, paranoia, seizures, coma

Neurotransmitter Effects of Amphetamines

- Increases release and blocks reuptake of natural catecholamines
  - Stimulates fight-or-flight effect
  - Dopamine and norepinephrine activation
  - Dopamine on basal ganglia: high-dose stereotype and aggression
  - Counterintuitive calming effects in ADD/ADHD

Signs and Symptoms of Intoxication

- Elevated blood pressure, heart rate, dysrhythmias
- Dilated pupils reactive to light
- Hyperactive tendon reflexes
- Shallow respiration
- Circulatory collapse
- Altered sensorium, hallucinations, paranoid feelings

Club Drug

- **MDMA (Ecstasy)** 3,4-Methylenedioxymethamphetamine
  - Combined w/other substances of abuse, such as:
  - Ingested and metabolized by liver
- Onset 30–60 minutes up to four hours
- "Crash" 4–12 hours after dose
- Post depression can last up to five days

Symptoms of Use and Hazards

- Muscle tension, teeth clenching
- Blurred vision, faintness, chills, sweating
- Confusion, neurocognitive functioning
- Depression, mood disturbances
- Sleep disorders, cardiovascular disorders
- Anxiety, paranoia
- Long-term memory impairment
- Parkinson's disease
- Eventual paralysis

Methamphetamine is a potent central nervous system stimulant that causes a rush of dopamine as well as norepinephrine and serotonin release when taken. As a legitimate medical prescription, it is a schedule II orally controlled drug by the name of **Desoxyn.** It is used to treat ADHD, narcolepsy, and obesity. It has a high addiction potential and is a drug that is considered dangerous.

As an illicit drug, it can be taken a number of ways: inhaled, snorted, orally, or anally. The onset of the euphoria a user experiences is felt within seconds or up to 15 minutes, depending on the method of administration. The neurotransmitter release from meth (especially dopamine) makes you feel euphoric, decreases appetite and fatigue, and increases alertness, well-being, and exhilaration. The mechanism of action is to stimulate the release of dopamine into the synaptic cleft. This will block the reuptake of dopamine and norepinephrine. Heavy use of methamphetamine often results in psychosis. Long-term methamphetamine use has been shown to cause changes in brain function and structure, impairing the monoamine system after chronic abuse. Meth will consume your entire existence.

Treatment of amphetamine-induced conditions includes initial treatment assessment with elimination of offending substance by gastric lavage, induced emesis, or charcoal. Selected medication treatment for amphetamine-induced disorders is varied. **Ammonium chloride (Quelidrine),** an OTC expectorant, has been found to acidify the urine, causing amphetamine excretion to increase.

Propranolol (Inderal), a beta-blocking antihypertensive, is useful in the treatment of anxiety, impulse control, and reduction of elevated blood pressure and pulse. **Naloxone (Narcan)** will reverse opioid effects in the event of concurrent opiate toxicity**. Lorazepam (Ativan)** and **chlordiazepoxide (Librium)** provide rapid, flexible sedation**. Haloperidol (Haldol),** a potent antipsychotic, dopamine antagonist, provides quick sedation of amphetamine-induced psychosis.

Methamphetamine crosses the placenta that feeds the fetus. The effects of the drug on the fetus are not fully understood. Meth may affect the fetus directly by transferring through the placenta or indirectly by changing the environment. Meth has **vasoconstrictive** effects, resulting in decreased **utero-placental** blood flow, causing the fetus to have high blood pressure and fetal hypoxia. This can result in prenatal stroke, heart malformations, and other organ damage in the fetus.

The condition of **preeclampsia** occurs in seemingly healthy women. When the mother has high blood pressure, she may have an edema level above normal. Preeclampsia may cause a woman to have a stroke or even die during her pregnancy or while giving birth. Methamphetamine can have the same effect as preeclampsia by elevating the blood pressure of the mother.

Women who use methamphetamine while pregnant can have premature labor. More than half the women in the United States who use meth through their pregnancy may not deliver full term. Meth babies born are underweight. Ten percent of women who use meth will suffer placental abruption. This is when the placenta prematurely detaches from the uterine wall before labor has begun. Babies who are born accustomed to meth will start withdrawals. The baby will often have problems feeding, with underdeveloped lungs and brain. The limited research information revealed outcomes of deficits in infant neurobehavioral function and growth problems when compared to other infants. Meth use is believed to have long-term effects on brain development, which may last for years. Children may have possible cognitive, language, motor, emotional, and behavioral problems when prenatally exposed to methamphetamine. Newborns exposed to meth often have sleep difficulties and problems with altered behavior. Once these children reach school age, they are known to be hyperactive or to have attention deficits, learning disabilities, and fits of anger.

The most common heart problems found in meth babies are **patent ductus arteriosus** (PDA) and low blood pressure. PDA is a persistent opening between two major blood vessels leading from the heart. This heart defect will often close by itself; however, it can have serious effects if it is left untreated. Untreated PDA can cause too much blood flow to the heart, and heart failure as well as other complications can occur.

Research conducted by the University of Toronto has found that a single use of crystal methamphetamine may cause neurodevelopment problems in babies. A developing fetus appears to be susceptible to DNA damage from exposure to methamphetamine in utero. The fetus's DNA is damaged because it has not yet developed the enzymes to protect it from free radicals. This susceptibility lasts from the embryonic stage through the later fetal stage when organs and mental function develops. An infant that is born to a methamphetamine-using mother is likely to have more severe brain abnormalities than an infant exposed to alcohol prenatally. A fetus that is exposed to both methamphetamine and alcohol may actually have even more severe, permanent damage (Smith, at el, 1149–1156).

The Infant Development, Environment, and Lifestyle Study (IDEAL) found lower growth rates in weight, height, and head circumference after birth in these methamphetamine-exposed infant groups compared to their unexposed infant peers. Infants exposed to methamphetamine prenatally are three and one-half times more likely to be small for their gestational age. This condition can lead to higher mortality rates and increased risk of developing type 2 diabetes. Fetal exposure to stimulants, such as cocaine and methamphetamine, has been shown to cause lower births and potential survival. (Smith, at el, 1149–1156)

One of the more troubling findings from The Infant Development, Environment, and Lifestyle Study (IDEAL) is the behavioral problems associated with children exposed to methamphetamine in the womb. Caregivers of methamphetamine-exposed children report an increase in signs of emotional instability, anxiety, and depression. The study found that this group of children shows high levels of decreased ability to sustain focus. Furthermore, caregivers are reporting aggressive and defiant behavior. Children who were exposed to methamphetamine prenatally are likely to be diagnosed with attention deficit hyperactivity disorder (ADHD) (Smith, at el, 1149–1156). This creates a crisis as the methamphetamine-exposed child grows older. Stimulants are often prescribed to treat ADHD diagnoses. An early introduction to stimulants, a high likelihood of aggression and defiance, problems with maintaining sustained focus, and having a mother that is/was a methamphetamine abuser creates the perfect combination for an individual to be susceptible to becoming a methamphetamine addict.

It must be noted that very few studies claim to have conclusive evidence on the effects of prenatal methamphetamine exposure on human test subjects. The majority of studies conducted on this subject have been performed using laboratory mice. Due to methamphetamine's relatively short half-life, testing a newborn infant for methamphetamine is not a definitive indicator of potential meth exposure during pregnancy. Researchers and doctors often rely on self-reporting by the mother to determine methamphetamine use. Again, this is an unreliable method of determining exposure.

Nicotine

Nicotine is derived from the tobacco plant. It is estimated that 5% of the tobacco plant contains nicotine. Nicotine is among the 4,000 chemicals found in the smoke of various tobacco products, which include pipes, cigars, and cigarettes. Research has revealed that despite the fact that there are thousands of chemicals in tobacco, nicotine is the only chemical that produces the feelings that draw people back to smoking. Nicotine addiction due to tobacco consumption is a major cause of disability and premature death. Demographically, tobacco addiction is higher in persons with mental illness and substance abuse disorders, which represent a high proportion of current smokers.

Administration is via inhalation (smoking tobacco and tars), intranasal (snuff), oral/buccal (chewing tobacco), oral/gastrointestinal (nicotine gum), and transcutaneous (patches). All forms produce comparable blood levels. There are no barriers to nicotine. The pharmacokinetics of nicotine is rapid, easy, quick absorption into the blood stream, and distribution throughout the whole body. This is the early rush to the brain. It is metabolized by the liver. Nicotine half-life is about two hours, after which physical and behavioral withdrawal can occur. Nicotine is as addictive as cocaine and heroin.

Nicotine pharmacodynamics is analogous to smoke. It distributes rapidly to all body compartments as well as the peripheral and central nervous system. Nicotine releases the neurotransmitters epinephrine, dopamine, and glutamate. It stimulates nicotinic acetylcholine receptors and enhances cortical activity, including attention and memory. This effect on **cortisol** appears to contribute to nicotine withdrawal. Activation of the reward pathway reinforces the desire to use the drug again. Nicotine binds to nicotinic cholinergic receptors, triggering neurotransmitter release, which affects multiple body systems. The neurotransmitters DA, NE, Glu, GABA, and 5-HT are working together to develop and maintain nicotine dependence and affect multiple layers of physiologic and psychological processes.

Nicotine Affects Multiple Neurotransmitters

- Dopamine, which may trigger the reward centers associated with the addictive properties.
- Norepinephrine, which may trigger the increase cardiovascular and arousal effects.
- Glutamate, which may trigger the enhancement of performance and cognition.
- GABA, which may trigger the sedative, calmness, and relaxation properties, and, on the other hand, the agitation during withdrawal.
- Serotonin, which may trigger the relaxing, antidepressant, and positive feelings.

Elevation of blood pressure, heart rate, and abnormal heart rhythms occur in the cardiovascular system. Nicotine increases the level of endorphins; they are a protein that is often referred to as a natural pain killer with a similar structure to morphine. This may be an indication of the psychoactive and rewarding effects of smoking. Additional nicotine effects are insulin sensitivity and insulin resistance. Smoking encourages mouth cancer, causes gum disease, and stains skin and teeth. Nicotine poisoning is a very common, with nicotine gum and "E-cigs." Pure nicotine is extremely poisonous and can cause death. Some of the long-term effects of smoking include sleeping disorders, irritability, poor concentration, severe headaches, and anxiety.

Nicotine's Effects on the Brain

- Behavior reinforcing action
- Vomiting and nausea tolerated rapidly
- Stimulates **hypothalamic antidiuretic hormone** and consequent fluid retention
- Reduces afferent input from muscles, lowering muscle tone
- Reduces weight gain by reducing appetite
- Increases blood flow to central nervous system causing:
  - Arousal, reward
  - Improves task performance
  - Antidepressant effect

Nicotine's Effects on the Body

- Tolerance
- Dependence
- Toxicity
- Diseases
  - Cardiovascular
  - Pulmonary
  - Cancer
- Infections
- Passive Smoke
- Pregnancy
  - Damages unborn children
- Environmental pollution

Top Five Reasons Why People Smoke

- It is a habit.
- I'm addicted.
- It relaxes me.
- I enjoy it.
- It gives me something to do with my hands.

Reasons Why Smokers Do Not Try to Quit

- Fear of withdrawal
- Cravings

Loss of way to handle stress

- Cost of medicines
- Fear cannot quit

Five Myths about Quitting Smoking

- Smoking is just a bad habit.
  - Fact: Tobacco use is an addiction.
- Quitting is just a matter of will power.
  - Fact: Quitting is difficult.
- If you can't quit the first time, you will never quit.
  - Fact: Quitting is hard and usually takes 2–3 tries.
  - (Quitting smoking may be a learned behavior: repeated failure may lead to success.)
- The best way to quit is "cold turkey."
  - Fact: The most effective way is a combination of counseling and nicotine replacement therapy.
- Quitting is expensive.
  - Fact: Treatments cost $3–14 per day. A pack-a-day smoker spends almost $1,200 per year. Many health insurance plans cover medication and counseling.

Pharmacotherapeutic approaches to tobacco addiction include nicotine replacement therapy (NRT), **bupropion, and varenicline**, the latter **a selective nicotine receptor partial agonist**.

Bupropion (Buspar, Zyban) dose is similar to that for the treatment of depression. Essentially, 100–150 mg of bupropion begins 1–2 weeks before the target quit date. Clinical trials have shown effectiveness for smoking cessation. Varenicline (Chantix) has been shown to reduce cravings and decrease the enjoyable effects of smoking. The side effect profile includes nausea, headache, and insomnia. Rare occurrences include thoughts of suicide, erratic behavior, and drowsiness, at which point, the drug is to be discontinued. Nicotine replacement therapy (NRT) includes nicotine gums, sprays, inhalers, patches, tablets, and lozenges. The advantage of NRT is that it's subject to strict quality control; however, it still comes with the inherent dangers of nicotine use. NRT safety in pregnancy has not been established. **Lobeline** is a naturally occurring alkaloid similar to nicotine. This agonist is used as a smoking cessation tool; however, there is currently no evidence to support its effect on abstinence.

Smoking Cessation

- Modify behavior and reward abstinence
  - Set a date, inform friends, family, and coworkers for understanding and support
- Avoid triggers
  - Remove cigarettes from environment and avoid places where smoking is prevalent
- Anticipate challenges
  - Critical first few weeks of withdrawal effects
  - Nicotine replacement and concurrent therapy

Nicotine Withdrawal

- Anxiety, frustration, irritability
- Impatience, restlessness
- Craving for tobacco
- Decreased blood pressure, heart rate, skin temperature
- Depression
- Gastrointestinal disturbances,
- Increased appetite, weight gain
- Headache, insomnia

Therapy for Nicotine Dependence

- Replacement (lozenges, patches and gum)
- Antidepressant
  - **Bupropion (Zyban, Wellbutrin)**
- **Chantix (Varenicline)**
  - **Partial agonist of nicotinic receptor** responsible for pleasurable nicotine effects
  - Stimulates dopamine release and reduces withdrawal symptoms
- Support: 1-800 NO BUTTS

Fetal Effects of Nicotine and Smoking

Nicotine and smoking expose the baby to an abundance of chemicals that increase risks to the unborn child. Compounds include carbon monoxide, styrene, vinyl chloride, formaldehyde, benzene, ammonia, lead, and others which restrict delivery of the oxygen and nutritional supply. This has negative effects on the small blood vessels of the placenta. The placenta is the organ responsible for bringing oxygen and nutrients from the mother to the baby.

When this tissue is exposed to toxins like nicotine, damage can be done—no matter how it is introduced to the body. Pregnancy-related health associations comprise placental complications, low birth weight, premature breaking of membranes, premature and stillborn births.

Babies exposed to nicotine and smoking have an increased risk of **sudden infant death syndrome (SIDS)** within the first year of life. Nicotine has been associated with childhood colic, asthma, respiratory difficulties, increased ear infections, allergies, and obesity. Some research suggests that smoking during pregnancy might affect a child's emotional development and behavior and ability to learn. Smoking during pregnancy may impair a child's own fertility. There is no safe level of smoking while pregnant. Nicotine crosses the **placental barrier** and interacts with the **endogenous acetylcholine receptors** in fetal brain and lungs. This exposure ,during development interferes with normal neurotransmitter function, subsequently evoking neurodevelopmental abnormalities by disrupting the timing of neural actions.

Nicotine can cause **ectopic (tubular) pregnancy**. Gastrointestinal disorders and facial disorders, cleft, lip, palate, heart defects, missing and deformed limbs or a clubfoot have been linked to nicotine use. Nicotine accumulates in breast milk, extending nicotine exposure during the postnatal period. The safety of nicotine replacement therapy has not been well documented. Health providers recommend complete abstinence from nicotine in any form during pregnancy to ensure the baby's health and safety. The growing popularity of "E-cigs" exposes the fetus to nicotine, fostering lowered birth weight and significant damage to the cardiovascular system; it is also one of the toxins implicated in placental damage. Some e-cigarette liquid tested contained traces of toxins, including cancer-causing chemicals like nitrosamines and formaldehyde.

Caffeine

Caffeine is a central nervous system stimulant found in plants, foods, drinks, and medications. The **United States Food and Drug Administration** classifies caffeine as both a food additive and a drug. Common sources are tea, cocoa, coffee, chocolate, and fortified mega drinks. Due to the influx of **high energy** drinks being sourced all over the world, there is concern over the proper dosage and toxicity levels of caffeine as well as its long-term health implications. It is consumed to obtain mild central nervous system stimulant effects and is the most widely used psychoactive substance leading to physical dependency.

Pharmacokinetics of caffeine is completely and rapidly absorbed from the gastrointestinal tract of humans with 99 percent of its absorption occurring within 45 minutes of ingestion (Caffeine for the Sustainment of Mental Task Performance, 2001). It follows **accumulation dosing**, meaning that prolonged used of caffeine through caffeinated beverages such as coffee has shown to increase tolerance levels and withdrawal symptoms in most individuals. This is thought to be due to the accumulation of paraxanthine concentration levels in the bloodstream. The half-life is about 5–6 hours (Csaijka, C. et al., 2005). It lasts longer late in pregnancy and in the elderly, is shorter in smokers, and concentrates in the breast milk.

Caffeine is metabolized in the liver and broken down into three metabolic dimethylxanthines. These include paraxanthine, theobromine, and theophylline. **Paraxanthin** breaks down fats, increases blood levels of glycerol and fats, and forms 84% of the metabolic dimethylxanthines. **Theobromine** dilates blood vessels and also has a diuretic effect, increasing urination and forming 12% of the metabolic dimethylxanthines. **Theophylline** dilates the airways and is used in the treatment of asthma; it forms 4% of the metabolic dimethylxanthines. These metabolites are further broken down and excreted in the urine (Ribeiro, J. A. and Sebastiao, A. M., 2010).

Pharmacodynamic effects in the cortex at normal doses (100–200 mg of caffeine) stimulate the rewarding effect, feelings of competency, alertness, sustained attention, faster thought, reduced fatigue, and lower need for sleep. Alternatively, fine motor coordination, timing accuracy, and arithmetic may be impaired. Heavy dosing (1.5 grams a day) may produce agitation, anxiety, tremors, panting, and insomnia. The mechanism of action has multiple layers. Caffeine travels through the bloodstream quickly and triggers a release of catecholamine, adrenaline, and noradrenaline (World of Caffeine 2015). It crosses the **blood-brain-barrier**, which is designed to separate the brain from the bloodstream. Once inside the brain, caffeine blocks the effects of adenosine. Specifically, **blockade of methylxanthine-sensitive adenosine receptors** is the currently accepted mechanism of action. A normal caffeine dose blocks 50% of adenosine receptors.

Adenosine is a neuromodulator linked to sleep-inducing effects, which play an important part in energy and sleep promotion. Adenosine and, thus, caffeine act on NE, DA, ACh , glutamate, and GABA neurotransmitters. This indirect stimulation of catecholamines causes elevation of blood pressure and heart rate (Ribeiro, J. A. and Sebastiao, A. M., 2010). Caffeine blocks GABA receptors, stimulates calcium release within the cells, and blocks adenosine receptors which result in behavioral stimulation. Additionally, it releases the hormones ghrelin (hunger), somatropin (growth), testosterone (sex), and cortisol (stress). Spinal cord stimulation occurs at toxic doses (2–5 grams), cardiac arrhythmias at 10–20 grams.

Pharmacotherapeutic use of caffeine is in combination with ergotamine for migraine headaches and in combination with nonsteroidal, anti-inflammatory drugs in analgesic formulations. Caffeine alone is used to promote wakefulness, to treat various headache conditions, respiratory depression in neonates, postprandial hypotension and obesity, and to enhance seizure duration in electroconvulsive therapy. In some headache and in pain models, caffeine may produce direct adjuvant analgesic properties, while in other headache conditions, caffeine may be effective by alleviating a manifestation of caffeine withdrawal. **Medicinal effects** contained in over-the-counter (OTC) stimulants include No-Doz 100 mg/tab and Vivarin 200 mg/tab. Caffeine has a synergistic interaction with analgesics, Anacin contains aspirin and 32 mg/tab of caffeine, Excedrin contains aspirin and 64.8 mg/tab of caffeine. Caffeine is found in OTC diuretics, cold preparations, and asthma and bronchodilation products.

The estimated average daily caffeine consumption among Americans is 280 mg per day. Many people think they are doing away with caffeine by drinking decaffeinated coffee. This is not true. **Decaffeinating** is a process, but in nine out of ten tested cups of decaffeinated coffee, there were still 8.6 mg to 13.9 mg of caffeine.

Caffeine Intake Levels

Low to moderate intake	130 mg to 300 mg per day
Moderate intake	200 mg to 300 mg per day
High intake	400 mg per day
Heavy intake	6,000 mg per day

Caffeine is considered addictive. The Diagnostic and Statistical Manual of Mental Disorders 4th edition lists the criteria for substance dependence as follows:

- Tolerance
- Substance-specific withdrawal syndrome
- Substance often taken in larger amounts over a longer period than expected
- Persistent desire or unsuccessful efforts to cut down or control use

- Time spent in activities to obtain, use, or recover from the effects of the substance
- Important activities given up or reduced because of substance
- Use continued despite knowledge of problems caused by substance

Caffeinism is a caffeine-induced disorder from DSM-IV. Patients show symptoms of caffeine tolerance, dependence, and withdrawal effects due to increased adenosine receptor density and, thus, increased adenosine sensitivity. At high doses >1000 mg/day, there are psychiatric effects.

The five caffeine-induced psychiatric disorders include caffeine intoxication, caffeine withdrawal, unspecified caffeine-related disorder, caffeine-induced anxiety disorder, and caffeine-induced sleep disorder.

Long-term use produces tolerance to some of the pharmacological effects. Discontinuation of regular caffeine use can present **caffeine withdrawal** even from moderate intake levels. This is characterized by headache, fatigue, anxiety, feeling less alert and less energetic, and experiencing difficulty concentrating. Discontinuing daily caffeine consumption produces changes in cerebral blood flow velocity and quantitative EEG that are likely related to the classic caffeine withdrawal symptoms of headache, drowsiness, and decreased alertness. More specifically, acute caffeine abstinence increased brain blood flow, an effect that may account for commonly reported withdrawal headaches. Acute caffeine abstinence also produced changes in EEG (increased theta rhythm) that has previously been linked to the common withdrawal symptom of fatigue. These symptoms usually last two to nine days but are individual in strength and length for each person.

Conflicting research is available for caffeine in pregnancy and effects on the fetus. Caffeine's ability to stimulate the heart can be dangerous to the fetus in pregnant women as there is no placental barrier to caffeine, causing it to be readily absorbed by the developing fetus. It is, therefore, recommended that pregnant women limit their intake of caffeine or avoid caffeine during pregnancy. Caffeine ingestion has been linked to low birth weight, premature delivery, and miscarriage. There is conflicting data on reproductive effects: it may slow growth *in utero*, especially in high doses, it may be harmful prior to conception, and it may increase the risk of spontaneous abortion.

Research on caffeine use is on adults. Its effect on children and adolescents are, as of now, still unknown. A research summary found in adults that caffeine is not:

- Associated with increases in blood pressure

- Linked to cardiovascular disease
- Has no scientific finding that it is harmful during pregnancy to mother or child or contributes to birth defects or fertility

However, research has found that caffeine consumption is associated with lower bone mineral density. It has also been found that caffeine contributes to weight gain by increasing stress hormones.

Alpha Omega

"My first realization that alcohol or drugs could have a negative impact on an individual's life is when I first realized that my mother was unable to participate in much of life without alcohol. I learned quickly the signs and behaviors of being intoxicated. Her addiction got worse, and I rebelled by putting a gap in our relationship. I told myself I would never be like her or, for that matter, any of my family. By the time I was in high school, I had used marijuana, smoked cigarettes, and drank to the point of blackouts. My mom entered her first attempt at treatment, and although I wanted to support her, I was angry and had fallen into the grip of meth (methamphetamine). To many people's surprise, I graduated high school loaded!

"After high school, I tried to stop using, only to switch addictions to coke (cocaine), ecstasy, and alcohol. I managed to hold on to a good job and go to school for a while. Eventually, I fell back into meth and a dysfunctional relationship which kept me loaded for the next four years.

"Eventually my addiction took over, I was introduced to the "dope game," and I lost my job and dropped out of school. I had many failed attempts to get clean and have a seminormal life without giving up the lifestyle or people. My life spiraled out of control, and I started stealing to support my habits! I had no coping skills; drug use was my only out.

"In 2012, I was taken off the streets and placed in the safest place for myself and others, jail. Even facing three felonies didn't making getting clean an option. I jumped at treatment as a way to get out of jail, with no intention of getting clean or leaving my dysfunctional relationship behind. As I spent the next eight months in custody, I started to get a little taste of recovery. My thoughts and actions were changing. When I finally went to treatment, everyone I thought was my friends disappeared, leaving me surrounded with people who only wanted me to succeed and get better! I would like to say that is when I surrendered. It took about five months of a six-month program for me to put both feet into my recovery.

"Now, a little over three and one-half years later, I can say that it was the best thing that ever happened to me! I found myself, my family, and my calling in life, which is to be a drug and alcohol counselor working with clients with co-occurring conditions. My life is now happier than I ever knew it could be, I have reestablished my relationships with my children, fell in love with my wife all over again, and am working as the assistant AOD counselor. I am finding it to be the most rewarding experience of my life! I never knew how sad my life was until I found true happiness!"—Anonymous

Critical Thinking

A young adult is going through turmoil in his or her life as his or her parents are getting divorced. He or she purchases **pseudoephedrine** because friends told him or her it gets them high. The teenager goes to the pharmacy and purchases the maximum amount of pseudoephedrine "behind the counter" that is allowed and takes much more than the recommended dosing amount to feel the effects of the drug. The teenager collapses of a cardiac arrhythmia.

For the above scenario, take a look at options, paths and outcomes of various choices. Use the Options for Thought below as a template for discussion, ideas and thought generation.

OPTIONS FOR THOUGHT

Remedy the situation by dealing with his or her emotions constructively.
Escapism, depression, feeling hopeless, reaching out.
School counselors, psychiatrist, support system; talking through.
Coping skills (healthy venting, exercise, natural high, reframe, etc.).

Addictive behavior pattern with no improvement in coping skills to deal with stressful situations.

Temporarily perceiving him or herself as being happy when in reality he or she is just high.

The teenager may end up getting into legal trouble, possibly even ending up in jail.

Review the Following Case Studies

CASE #1

Athletes use and abuse **ephedrine** for the weight loss and performance enhancing benefits. There is evidence that the pressure on young athletes to perform and to outperform their competitors is so great that many are risking their lives with dietary supplements. These over-the-counter products are not regulated by the government and may contain powerful and dangerous ingredients. In 2002 (source CNS News), Rashidi Wheeler was a driven player and a rising star of the Northwestern University football team. His sudden death at practice raised questions. The preliminary cause of death was listed as bronchial asthma, but teammates reportedly say Wheeler may have taken a performance enhancer that contains the stimulant ephedrine. Dozens of supplements on store shelves contain it, and it's legal. The supplements promise to increase stamina and cut weight, but many physicians say they simply trick the body—with sometimes deadly consequences. The Food and Drug Administration has reports of at least 80 deaths associated with products containing ephedrine, but an industry group says it is safe.

Case #2

Imagine a 23-year-old white woman. She weighs 108 pounds and she is 5′8″. She is smoking **methamphetamine** in an abandoned suburban home at 3 a.m. This woman has been getting high with a low-level meth dealer for the past five days. The pair, like many meth users, have unprotected sex when they are high (Zapata, LB, et al. 641–648). She notices that she has not menstruated in at least six weeks. The last thing on her mind is the possibility of a pregnancy. She has just broken into a car and is looking for someone to buy or trade her newly acquired, stolen laptop. She is in need of some more meth and a pack of cigarettes. At five months, she is barely showing signs of her pregnancy. She has not bothered to go to the doctor. She plans on "doing that in a couple of days." Halfway through the third trimester, she only weighs 124 pounds. The fetus in her womb does not get any nutrients because his mother hardly ever eats. The little baby boy is born three weeks early, and he is grossly underweight.

Case #3

Mikes' mother used **amphetamines and cocaine** during her pregnancy. He was born underweight, with a small bone structure, underdeveloped organs, and numerous respiratory problems. The effects of his mother's stimulant use have become more severe as Mike got older. Mike suffers from attention deficit hyperactivity disorder, depression, anxiety, and polysubstance abuse disorder. He became addicted to methamphetamine at the age of 12 years old. The physical effects of his prenatal exposure to stimulants are possibly the least harmful aspect of this situation. "Growing up as the child of a mother who was addicted to methamphetamine has had a much more devastating effect on my overall ability to function normally," he says.

Case #4

"I have a 14-year-old, and I am not proud of this, but I used **meth** my entire pregnancy. As a result of that, he is developmentally delayed. He didn't walk until he was 19 months old; he has done everything later than the average child. He can be very aggressive ,at times, and unpredictable. He is a year behind in school and has to be in a special day class. He has a diagnosed processing disorder as well as bipolar disorder. Austin struggles to make and keep friends and pretty much just stays in his room. So if there is any doubt that meth causes long-term effects in a child that has been exposed while inside the womb, please let me be the one to tell you there are long-term effects; I see them in my own child every day."—Anonymous

Case #5

"In my early twenties, a neighbor gave me my first line of **meth**, and I was hooked from that moment. The rush and the high were just too good. I remember it also making me feel like I was invincible and no longer felt insecure. A few years later, I added alcohol to the mix. My disease of addiction was in full bloom. I managed to stay functioning until my late 30s. The consequences were stacking up, and my life was falling apart. My consistently bad choices had finally lead to losing everything except the roof over my head. I was mentally at my breaking point, and my health was very bad. I hit my bottom facedown, there was nowhere left to go but up or dead."—Anonymous

WISH

Overview of Psychoactive Drugs:

https://www.youtube.com/watch?v=icD3l5bhhKY

Psychoactive Drugs: Stimulants:

https://www.youtube.com/watch?v=1Smz0zwAELQ

Cocaine

Cocaine in the Human Brain:

https://www.youtube.com/watch?v=Tqwo9dmIXAQ

Amphetamines

Amphetamine Anatomy:

https://www.youtube.com/watch?v=_Jlivz3xsUE

Neurotransmitters and Amphetamines:

https://www.youtube.com/watch?v=Ju_qha2OBL4

Amphetamines Overview:

https://www.youtube.com/watch?v=fEyEsxzeqWo

Brain on MDMA:

https://www.youtube.com/watch?v=jEAr7ThsYew

Methamphetamine

Meth Inside and Out:

https://www.youtube.com/watch?v=w98Fn8JofCw

The World's Most Dangerous Drug:

https://www.youtube.com/watch?v=at3Sg6qvgTE

Nicotine

Nicotine Animation:

https://www.youtube.com/watch?v=2L8ZkbtEv3E

How Smoking Affects the Body:

https://www.youtube.com/watch?v=SwYEFu-GKP4

Nicotine Withdrawal Video:

https://www.youtube.com/watch?v=HlcIKekEldg

Caffeine

How Caffeine Affects Your Brain:

https://www.youtube.com/watch?v=P8ToQQLAIU8

Adenosine: Brain on Coffee:

https://youtu.be/4YOwEqGykDM

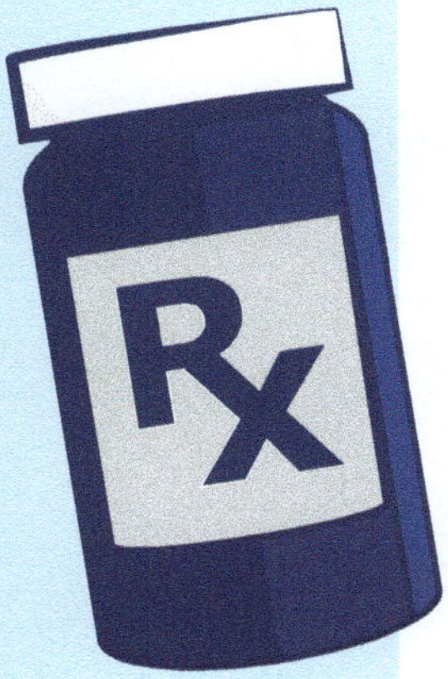

Drug Sandbox

IMPORTANT WORDS TO KNOW!

Speed
Thermogenesis
Decongestant
Appetite Suppressant
Concentration Booster
Methamphetamine
Amphetamines
Indirect Catecholamine Agonist
Ammonium Chloride (Quelidrine®)
Propranolol (Inderal®)
Naloxone (Narcan®)
Lorazepam (Ativan®)
Chlordiazepoxide (Librium®)
Haloperidol (Haldol®)
Pseudoephedrine
DAWN
Butyrylcholinesterase (BChE
Cocaethylene
Enzoylecgonine
Placental Abruption
Diazepam
Haloperidol,
Propranolol
Cocaine Antagonist
Dopamine Agonists
Bupropion
Imipramine
Dopamine Antagonist
Disulfiram (Antabuse®)
Buprenorphine
Nepicastat
Benzodiazepine
Valium
Xanax,
Antidepressants
Vigabatrin
Modafinil
Tiagabine
Topiramate
Cocaine Vaccine
Behavioral Treatments
Attention Deficit Disorder and Attention Deficit Hyperactivity Disorder
Sympathomimetic
Psychostimulant
MDMA (Ecstasy)
Methamphetamine
Desoxyn
Uteroplacental
Preeclampsia
Vasoconstrictive
Patent Ductus Arteriosus
Nicotine Pharmacodynamics
Cortisol
Hypothalamic Antidiuretic Hormone
Pharmacotherapeutic Approaches to Tobacco Addiction
Bupropion
Selective Nicotine Receptor Partial Agonist
Lobeline
Bupropion (Zyban®, Wellbutrin®)
Chantix (Varenicline®)
Partial Agonist of Nicotinic Receptor
Fetal Effects of Nicotine and Smoking
Sudden Infant Death Syndrome (SIDS)

Placental Barrier
Endogenous Acetylcholine Receptors
Ectopic (Tubular) Pregnancy
United States Food and Drugs Administration
High Energy Drinks
Paraxanthine
Theobromine
Theophylline
Blood-brain Barrier
Blockade of Methylxanthine-Sensitive Adenosine Receptors
Adenosine Neuromodulator
Medicinal Effects
Decaffeinating
Caffeinism
Caffeine withdrawal

Community Connections

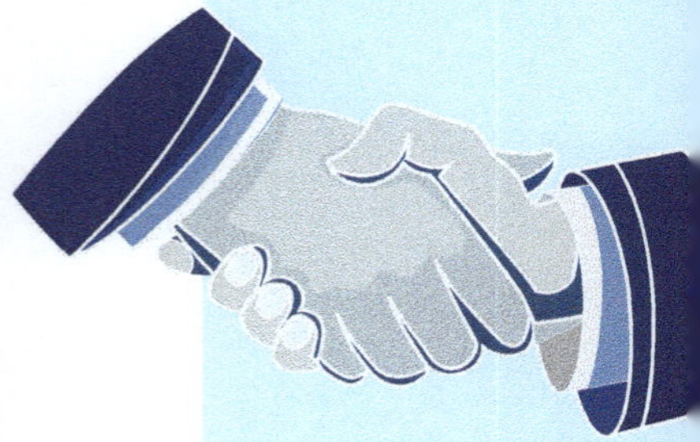

FIELD NOTES AND ANALYSIS: FOOD ADDICTS IN RECOVERY ANONYMOUS

"Food Addicts in Recovery Anonymous (FA) meetings are near my home. The meeting schedule indicated that the meeting on Tuesday nights at 7 p.m. is open to the public. Upon arrival at the meeting location, I noticed that many of the cars that were arriving were newer, high-priced vehicles. I rechecked the address for the meeting. I was in the right place. I walked through a set of double doors and entered a hallway that led to the main room. I began looking around the room to see if there were any signs indicating what type of building I was entering. No signage could be found. A table was set up on the left side of the room with FA literature and pamphlets. I started gathering a few pamphlets for future reading, then noticed the pamphlets had a price written on them. I had forgotten to grab cash before I came to the meeting. I put the pamphlets down.

"I scanned the room to evaluate the environment. Approximately 50 chairs were arranged in a half-moon shape. The focal point of the seating arrangement was a table in the center of the room. One chair was set up behind the table. The interior of the room was constructed of beautiful hardwood. I'm not an expert on hardwood, so I do not know what type it was. The ceiling had the same hardwood construction as the walls. There was a white piece of fabric draped lengthwise in the middle of the ceiling. In the far corner of the room, there was a stage and something covered with a sheet. I believe that it may have been an organ or piano.

"At the time of my arrival, there was only about 10–15 people in the room. I surveyed the seating arrangement to find the ideal seat to observe the meeting and its attendees. A seat in the back row and off to the side would give me the best vantage point to see the person sitting at the front table and observe the people sitting in the audience. Within one minute of sitting down, I was asked if this was the first time I had been to a meeting. I told the man that it was, in fact, my first FA meeting. He informed me that it is requested that 'we' sit in the first three rows. I apologized and introduced myself, 'Hi, my name is Jack and I am observing your meeting for a college assignment that I am doing. May I ask you a few questions?'

"The man introduced himself as Rudy. Rudy is in his fifties, approximately the same height as me with a moderately-sized belly on him. Rudy told me the building we are in is a Jewish synagogue, and it is set up with a special seating arrangement because the congregation is celebrating a Jewish holiday. He said there are normally less seats set up for FA. I asked Rudy what brought him to FA. He explained that he has 29 years of sobriety in Alcoholics Anonymous (AA), and he has been doing the FA program for three years. He reports that he lost almost 100 pounds when he was diligent about sticking to his sponsor-prescribed meal plan. He said that he stopped going to meetings for five months because he believed he 'could do it on his own.' With a look of shame on his face, he discloses that he 'gained about 50 pounds in five months.' He explained that sugar and flour are the drugs in FA.

"I sat down in the third row, and Rudy sat behind me. I thought we were supposed to be sitting in the front three rows? I thought to myself, 'Was he sitting behind me to keep an eye on the outsider?' I heard a voice coming through a speaker system, 'Welcome to the meeting of Food Addicts in Recovery Anonymous. My name is Peter, and I am a food addict.' Peter announced that the group asks people in their first 90 days of abstinence to raise their hands so they can be selected to come to the front of the room to recite the readings. Peter then welcomed everyone in attendance to join him in saying the Serenity Prayer. After the prayer, I did a thorough scan of the meeting attendees. I expected to see grossly overweight people wearing running shoes, but I observed something very different. Mostly everyone was older, white, and nicely dressed. I only noticed one woman wearing activewear clothing.

The majority of the people in attendance had grey hair and were unusually underweight!

"It was apparent that most of the people were from the middle class or upper class. To my surprise, many people were very skinny. There were a handful of extremely obese attendees. It was a balanced ratio of men and women. As I was observing the crowd of 50 people that had filled the room, I noticed many people were looking at me with curiosity. I had to tell myself not to squirm in discomfort. I knew that they knew that I was not one of them. Peter picked a different person for each of the program's formal readings. There were approximately 15 different readings that outlined everything we should know about the FA Program: Who is a food addict? What is the FA Program? How it Works. The 12 Traditions. The Clarity Statement (distinguishing that FA members identify themselves as food addicts). Another reading asked people to not talk about specific foods. I noted that FA reads their 12 Steps directly from the AA Big Book and did not replace the word Alcoholic with Food Addict.

"An older woman stood up in the crowd and announced that she was the secretary of that the meeting as well as the general service representative for the group. I was a bit surprised that she was sitting with the crowd as opposed to sitting where Peter was sitting. Other 12-Step fellowship meetings are facilitated by the secretary of meeting at the front of the room. It appears that the speaker for the night was the person who facilitates the group. Peter then announced, 'The Seventh Tradition states that each group is self-supported, and donations are not required for membership, but they are appreciated because rent for this facility is high.' Two baskets were passed around the room. People were dropping $1 or $5 bills in the baskets. They didn't pass the basket to me.

"Peter stood up and handed a laminated blue poster to a woman sitting in the front row. I could see two pictures of an obese man on the poster. With a microphone in in his hand, Peter announced, 'I'm Peter, and I am a food addict.' He spoke with a heavy German accent. Peter told the group that he was born in Germany during WWII. He described his dysfunctional, alcoholic family and the trauma he experienced growing up in a volatile home. Peter spoke of the unmanageability in his life that was the result of an addictive personality. He reported that he had numerous obesity-related health problems and was on mood stabilizers when he came to FA. He announced to the group that he just celebrated three years of abstinence in FA. He proudly announced that he is at 151 lbs, down from 265 lbs.

"Peter spoke with gratitude to his sponsor for creating a rigidly structured plan to help him lose the obsession to eat flour and sugar. It was touching when Peter expressed his gratitude for Bill W. (the founder of Alcoholics Anonymous) for creating the 12 Steps. Peter also explained that much of his growth came from Another Way of Life (AWOL) step-working groups. Peter finished by thanking his higher power for saving his life. Peter spoke for 30 minutes. The poster that Peter circulated had two pictures of himself before he came into recovery, one at 261 lbs and another at 257 lbs. Peter sat down after his share and delivered a few more announcements. He asked anyone with less than 90 days of abstinence to raise his or her hands. He asked the group's newcomer greeters to please stand. Peter then instructed everyone who is new to the program to speak with the newcomer greeters during the break.

"I approached Peter during the break and introduced myself as a student researcher. I asked him to provide me with specifics about how the FA Program works. He explained to me that abstinence is defined as not eating foods containing sugar and flour. He said that FA works by following a very rigid meal plan consisting of three meals a day. Each meal is comprised of 6 oz of protein, 6 oz of cooked vegetables, and 10 oz of uncooked vegetables. Each portion must be weighed using a digital scale. Every night, a member calls another member to make a commitment about the specific food they each plan to eat the next day. A member's sponsor prescribes specific foods that are acceptable to be included in each meal. I asked Peter to explain the AWOL meetings to me. AWOL is a closed group where members work their 12 Steps together. Peter's AWOL group has 150 members and meets every week in San Rafael. This is different than other 12-Step fellowships that work their steps like AA or Narcotics Anonymous. Members work their steps privately with their sponsor. FA members work each step as a group.

"Peter made the announcement that the meeting was now open for sharing but clarified that only members with 90 days of continuous recovery can share with the group. He called on five members to come to the front of the room one by one. Each shared his or her recovery story for five minutes. Each member started his or her share with his or her pre-recovery height and weight, then provided his or her current height and weight. The average weight loss for all of the speakers was around 100 lbs. The youngest member in the meeting was a 35-year-old woman who weighs 123 lbs. She reports that she weighed 233 lbs when she came into recovery. Every speaker mentioned that he or she needed the structure that the program provided. The highlight of the stories that I heard was when a woman described her experience at the FA camp out the previous weekend. She said the lines to get food took 'forever' because each person had to weigh out his or her portions. The group laughed in agreement when she mentioned that the caterers said they 'had never seen plates be so clean after being eaten off of.' The meeting was closed with the Serenity Prayer.

"I made my way to my car and jotted down my notes. A few thoughts:

- If addiction is considered by many as an obsessive-compulsive disorder, isn't religiously weighting one's food obsessive and compulsive?
- The rigid structure and formality of FA seem to go against 12-Step principles of letting go, acceptance, and turning one's will over to God.
- Why are newcomers not allowed to speak in meetings? That seems to be the opposite of 'principles before personalities' and anonymity." —Jack

End Of Chapter Review Questions

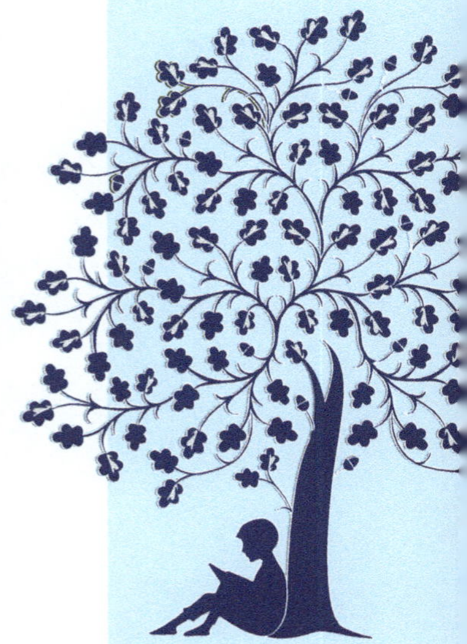

Matching: Using the list below, select the best answer:

a.	Ephedrine	1.	Analogous to smoke, it distributes rapidly to all body compartments, releasing epinephrine, dopamine, and glutamate. Its effect on cortisol appears to contribute to withdrawal.
b.	Cocaine	2.	Found in over-the-counter products as an herbal stimulant, it is available for symptomatic relief of asthma attacks, shortness of breath, chest tightness, and as a bronchodilator and decongestant.
c.	Amphetamines	3.	As a legitimate drug by the name of Desoxyn, this potent central nervous

			system stimulant causes a rush of dopamine, norepinephrine, and serotonin release when taken.
d.	Methamphetamine	4.	Common sources are tea, cocoa, coffee, chocolate, and fortified mega drinks. It is a central nervous system stimulant found in plants, foods, drinks, and medications; it is classified by the FDA as both a food additive and a drug.
e.	Nicotine	5.	The alcohol abstinence treatment, disulfiram (Antabuse), has produced the most consistent reductions in this drug's abuse.
f.	Caffeine	6.	MDMA (ecstasy) is from this pharmacologic therapeutic classification.

Multiple Choices: Select the best answer from the choices given:

7. Release of _______ may explain the addictiveness of nicotine.
    a. Norepinephrine
    b. Serotonin
    c. Dopamine
    d. GABA

8. Which of the following best describes the mechanism of action of cocaine?
    a. GABA agonist
    b. Monoamine reuptake inhibitor
    c. Beta blocker
    d. Dopamine antagonist

9. Which of the following neurotransmitters increase with amphetamine use?
    a. Dopamine
    b. Norepinephrine
    c. Serotonin
    d. All of the above

10. Which of the following is an element of smoking cessation therapy?

a. Behavior modification
b. Rewarding abstinence
c. Avoiding triggers
d. Removing cigarettes from the environment
e. All of the above

11. Which of the following appear(s) to have cocaine antagonizing or blocking effects?
    a. Diazepam
    b. Haloperidol
    c. Propranolol
    d. Only A and C
    e. All of the above

12. Discontinuation of regular caffeine use can present caffeine withdrawal even from moderate intake levels. This is characterized by all of the following except:
    a. Headache
    b. Fatigue
    c. Anxiety
    d. Alertness
    e. Difficulty concentrating

13. Common side effects of ephedrine that are similar to those produced by amphetamines include all of the following except:
    a. Calmness
    b. Insomnia
    c. Tremor
    d. Nervousness
    e. Restlessness

14. ________ plays a role in placental abruption.
    a. Caffeine
    b. Cocaine
    c. Theophylline
    d. Chantix
    e. Xanax

15. All of the following can be used in the treatment of amphetamine-induced disorders except:
    a. Ammonium chloride (Quelidrine)
    b. Propranolol (Inderal)
    c. Naloxone (Narcan)
    d. Lorazepam (Ativan)
    e. Methamphetamine (Desoxyn)

16. Symptoms of amphetamine use might be indistinguishable from _______.
    a. Heroin
    b. Nicotine
    c. Caffeine
    d. Pseudoephedrine
    e. Cocaine

17. Symptoms of use and hazards associated with MDMA use include:
    a. Problems with neurocognitive function
    b. Mood disturbances
    c. Heart arrhythmias
    d. All of the above

18. Caffeine effects can cause:
    a. Excitement and restlessness
    b. Tremors and anxiety
    c. Gastrointestinal disturbances
    d. All of the above

19. Treatment for amphetamine-induced psychosis includes:
    a. Haloperidol
    b. Nicotine
    c. Caffeine
    d. Diazepam
    e. Varenicline

Indicate if the following statement is true (A) or false (B):

20. Lobeline affects the brain in a similar way to nicotine and is used for smoking cessation.

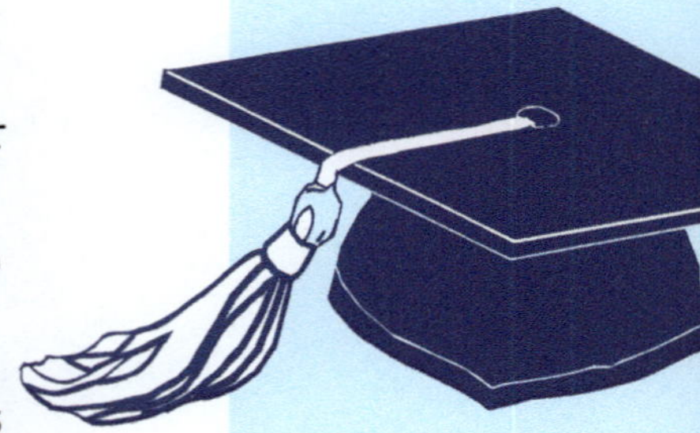

Applications: Assessment of Usage and Relevance

1. How can we treat nicotine addiction? Explain, with examples, the various methods used in the treatment of nicotine addiction. What factors contribute to the success of relapse prevention?

2. Describe the pharmacodynamics of nicotine, outlining the side effects. Since nicotine is now known to act to enhance dopamine activity in the nucleus accumbens, should it be reclassified as an amphetamine like cocaine? Why or why not?

3. Explain the pharmacokinetics and pharmacodynamics of caffeine and the mechanism responsible for caffeinism and withdrawal.

4. How do the effects of amphetamines change with increasing dosage? Why are they paradoxically effective in treating ADD/ADHD?

5. Analyze why powdered cocaine HCl is popular with the upper middle class, and why crack cocaine use is epidemic in inner city neighborhoods.

6. Evaluate the research on crack babies.

7. What is the pharmacodynamics of cocaine? What are its short-term- and long-term side effects?

8. How does tolerance to cocaine develop?

9. What are the various methods for administering nicotine? What are the relative blood levels produced by each method? Explain the advantages and disadvantages of the various routes of administration of nicotine.

KEY

1. E	6. C	11. E	16. C
2. A	7. F	12. D	17. D
3. D	8. B	13. A	18. D
4. F	9. D	14. B	19. A
5. B	10. E	15. E	20. A

REFERENCES

Ephedrine

Food and Drug Administration. "Dietary Supplements Containing Ephedrine Alkaloids; Proposed Rule." Federal Register (1997).

Journal. NAMSDL. 31 December 2013.

Paul G. Shekelle, et al. Efficacy and Safety of Ephedra and Ephedrine for Weight Loss and Athletic Performance: A Meta-analysis. 26 March 2003.

Stores, National Association of Chain Drug. State-By-State PSE Summaries. 2010.

WebMD. Drugs and Medications Ephedrine.

http://www.drugs.com/pro/ephedrine-sulphate-injection.html.

http://www.vanderbilt.edu/AnS/psychology/health_psychology/Ephedrine_wtloss.htm.

http://www.drugs.com/pseudoephedrine.html.

http://www.drugs.com/ephedrine.html.

http://www.narconon.org/drug-abuse/prescription/pseudoephedrine.html.

http://www.cbsnews.com/news/football-players-death-linked-to-ephedrine/.

Cocaine

Web MD. (2015). Drug use and pregnancy. Retrieved September 6, 2015, from Web MD website: http://www.webmd.com/baby/drug-use-and-pregnancy.

Gorski, T. T. (2002, March 5). Cocaine use during pregnancy. Retrieved September 4, 2015, from The Addiction website of Terence T. Gorski: http://www.tgorski.com/Prevention/cocaine_use_during_pregnancy.html.

Derlet R. W., Albertson T. E., and Rice P. Antagonism of cocaine, amphetamine, and methamphetamine toxicity.

http://www.nlm.nih.gov/medlineplus/druginfo/meds/a682602.html.

http://www.ncbi.nlm.nih.gov/pubmed/2217500.

http://www.drugabuse.gov/publications/research-reports/cocaine/what-treatments-are-effective-cocaine-abusers.

www.drugabuse.gov.

www.teens.drugabuse.gov.

http://www.drugaddictiontreatment.com/types-of-addiction/cocaine-types-of-addiction/disulfiram-for-cocaine-abuse/.

Substance Abuse and Mental Health Services Administration Health Information Network: www.store.samhsa.gov.

Methamphetamine

Zapata, L. B., et al. "Methamphetamine Use Is Independently Associated With Recent Risky Sexual Behaviors And Adolescent Pregnancy." Journal Of School Health 78.12 (2008): 641–648. CINAHL Complete. Web. 13 Sept. 2015.

Prah, Pamela M. Methamphetamine. [Electronic Resource]. n.p.: Washington, D.C. : CQ Press, 2005., 2005. SRJC Library Catalog. Web. 13 Sept. 2015.

Dyk, Jessie van, et al. "Maternal Methamphetamine Use In Pregnancy And Long-Term Neurodevelopmental And Behavioral Deficits In Children." Journal Of Population Therapeutics And Clinical Pharmacology = Journal De La Thérapeutique Des Populations Et De La Pharamcologie Clinique 21.2 (2014): e185-e196. MEDLINE with Full Text. Web. 13 Sept. 2015.

"Study: Just One Hit Of Meth Harms Fetuses." UPI Newstrack (Consumer Health) (2005): Consumer Health Complete—EBSCOhost. Web. 13 Sept. 2015.

Smith, L. M., LaGasse, L. L., Derauf, C., Grant, P., Shah, R., Arria, A., Huestis, M., Haning, W., Strauss, A., Della Grotta, S., Liu, J., and Lester, B. M. (2006). The Infant Development, Environment, and Lifestyle Study: Effects of Prenatal Methamphetamine Exposure, Polydrug Exposure, and Poverty on Intrauterine Growth. Pediatrics, 118(3), 1149–1156. doi: 10.1542/peds.2005-2564.

Chandler, Kelly. (FEB.2010). Prenatal Methamphetamine Exposure: The Child Effects.

Hackathorn, Cynthia. (2010). Multidimensional functioning in children with prenatal methamphetamine exposure.

LaGasse, Linda, Wouldes, Trecia, Newman, Elana, and Smith, Lynne. (6 July 2010). Prenatal methamphetamine exposure and neonatal behavioral outcome in USA and New Zealand.

McGuinness, Tina, and Daniel Pollack. (May 2008). Parental Methamphetamine Abuse and Children New Mother fact sheet: Methamphetamine use during pregnancy. North Dakota Department of Health. (Retrieved Oct. 2011).

"Fetal Development Timeline." BabyCenter. Web. 22 Aug. 2015. http://www.babycenter.in/a1050220/fetal-development-timeline.

"Latest In Recovery." Drug Abuse Alternatives Center (DAAC) Perinatal Day Treatment in Santa Rosa, California. Web. 24 Aug. 2015.

"Premature Birth." Complications. Web. 22 Aug. 2015. http://www.mayoclinic.org/diseases-conditions/premature-birth/basics/complications/CON-20020050.

"Risk and Reality: The Implications of Prenatal Exposure to Alcohol and Other Drugs." ASPE. 13 June 2015. Web. 22 Aug. 2015.

"What Are the Effects of Crystal Meth on Pregnancy?" LoveToKnow. Web. 22 Aug. 2015. .http://Crystalmethaddiction.org.

National Institute on Drug Abuse (NIH) June 1, 2008.

Nicotine

Griffin, R. Morgan. "E-Cigarettes 101." WebMD Smoking Cessation Health Center. WebMD,3Jan.2014.Web.14Sept.2015.http://www.webmd.com/smoking-cessation/features/electronic-cigarettes.

"Is It Safe to Use E-cigarettes While I'm Pregnant?" BabyCenter. BabyCenter, Nov. 2013. Web. 14 Sept. 2015. http://www.babycentre.co.uk/x25008139/is-it-safe-to-use-e-cigarettes-while-im-pregnant.

Mayo Clinic staff. "Smoking and Pregnancy: Understand the Risks." Mayo Foundation for Medical Education and Research. Mayo Clinic, 19 Mar. 2015. Web. 14 Sept. 2015. http://www.mayoclinic.org/healthy-lifestyle/pregnancy-week-by-week/in-depth/smoking-and-pregnancy/art-20047021.

Pagano, Trina, ed. "Effects of Smoking During Pregnancy." WebMD Health & Pregnancy Center. WebMD, 30 May 2014. Web. 14 Sept. 2015. http://www.webmd.com/baby/smoking-during-pregnancy.

"Tobacco Use and Pregnancy." Centers for Disease Control and Prevention, 5 Aug. 2014. Web. 14 Sept. 2015. http://www.cdc.gov/reproductivehealth/tobaccousepregnancy/.

Centers for Disease Control and Prevention., 05 Aug. 2014. Web. 18 Aug. 2015. http://www.cdc.gov/reproductivehealth/tobaccoUsePregnancy/index.htm.

Chasnoff, Ira J. "E-cigarette Use in Pregnancy." Psychology Today. n.p., n.d. Web. 18 Aug. 2015. https://www.psychologytoday.com/blog/aristotles-child/201404/e-cigarette-use-in-pregnancy.

"Pregnancy Week by Week." Smoking and Pregnancy: Understand the Risks. n.p., n.d. Web. 18 Aug. 2015. http://www.mayoclinic.org/healthy-lifestyle/pregnancy-week-by-week/in-depth/smoking-and-pregnancy/art-20047021.

"Tobacco Use and Pregnancy." Centers for Disease Control and Prevention, 05 Aug. 2014. Web. 18 Aug. 2015. http://www.cdc.gov/reproductivehealth/tobaccoUsePregnancy/index.htm.

Caffeine

Caffeine for the Sustainment of Mental Task Performance: Formulations for Military Operations. (Institute of Medicine (US) Committee on Military Nutrition Research, Comp.). (2001). Washington, D.C, U.S: National Academies Press. http://www.ncbi.nlm.nih.gov/books/NBK223808/.

Csajka, C., Haller, C. A., Benowitz, N. L., and Verotta, D. (2005). Mechanistic pharmacokinetic modelling of ephedrine, norephedrine and caffeine in healthy subjects. British Journal Of Clinical Pharmacology, 59(3), 335–345.

Ribeiro, J. A., and Sebastião, A. M. (2010). Caffeine and Adenosine. Journal Of Alzheimer's Disease, 203–15. doi:10.3233/JAD-2010-1379.

Smit, H. J., Cotton, J. R., Hughes, S. C., and Rogers, P. J. (2004). Mood and cognitive performance effects of "energy" drink constituents: caffeine, glucose and carbonation. Nutritional Neuroscience, 7(3), 127–139.

Thorn, Caroline F, Aklillu, Eleni, McDonagh, Ellen M., Klein, Teri E., and Altman, Russ B. "PharmGKB summary: caffeine pathway." Pharmacogenetics and genomics (2012). Retrieved on 12/08/15. Website: https://www.pharmgkb.org/pathway/PA165884757.

Brain, Marshall, Charles W. Bryant, and Matt Cunningham. HowStuffWorks. HowStuffWorks.com. n.d. Web. 12 Dec. 2015.

"Caffeine & Neurotransmitters." World of Caffeine. n.p., n.d. Web. 12 Dec. 2015.

Kalumuck, Karen E., PhD. "Caffeine." Salem Press Encyclopedia of Science. n.p.: Salem, 2015. Web. 12 Dec. 2015.

Nehlig, Astrid. "Caffeine and Headache." Nutrition, Brain and Behavior: Coffee, Tea, Chocolate, and the Brain (2004)

http://medicinenet.com/caffeine/article.htm.

http://coffeetea.about.com.

www.webmd.com.

www.drugs.com.

CHAPTER FIVE

DEPRESSANTS

Chapter Objectives

1. Outline the classification of depressants and the drugs.
2. List the mechanism of action of each depressant.
3. Characterize the essential signs and symptoms of each depressant drug usage, overdose, and withdrawal effects.

Positive Affirmations

"The thing we surrender to becomes our power."

—Ernest Holmes

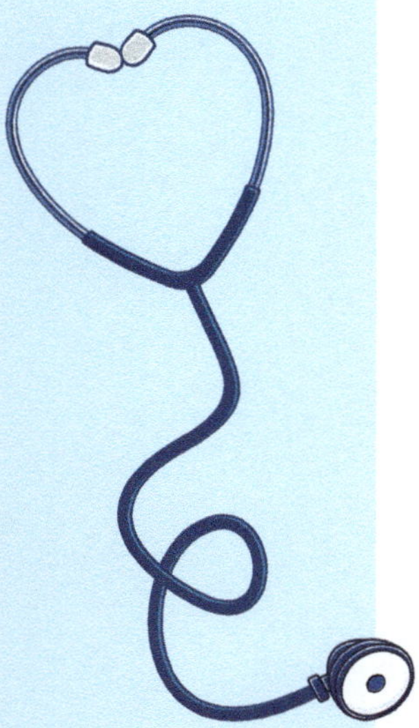

Pharmacology

Alcohol

Alcohol is classified as a depressant and anesthetic. It contains the components ethyl alcohol or ethanol ingredients found in medicines, beer, wine, and liquor and are a product of fermentation by yeast, sugars, and starches. For systemic effect, many cough and mouthwash products contain up to 25% or 50 proof of alcohol with the addition of antihistamines on board! Ethyl alcohols' local effect can be used topically as a germicide, irritant, and astringent.

Pharmacokinetics of ethanol involves oral administration and 80% absorption from the upper intestine. The rate limiting factor is the speed of stomach emptying; however, total absorption is unaffected by food. Once alcohol is absorbed by the stomach, it distributes to every tissue with over 90% access to all body compartments affecting every organ. Alcohol is converted by alcohol dehydrogenase to acetaldehyde. Acetaldehyde is converted by aldehyde dehydrogenase to acetic acid then to CO_2 and water. Metabolism is via the liver with 95% of alcohol metabolized by alcohol dehydrogenase enzyme and cytochrome P450. The liver accounts for 85% of alcohol metabolism; the balance is eliminated via lungs and kidneys. All women, alcoholic or not, have 60% less stomach alcohol dehydrogenase than men. Therefore, women appear to be even more vulnerable than men to intoxication and chronic effects.

The pharmacodynamics of ethanol is dependent on a variety of factors, including a person's size, weight, age, and sex, as well as the amount of food and alcohol consumed. Alcohol affects millions of nerve cells and changes communication patterns throughout the brain by slowing brain synapse firing, which alters and disrupts normal cell chemical behavior. Alcohol inhibits glutamate release and action at the receptors, increases glutamate release during withdrawal as an excitotoxic, and acts as a GABA and dopamine agonist (stimulator!). Glutamate-NMDA receptor is affected by alcohol with the most intensity. The result is a super-sized combination of DA positive and GABA negative reinforcement.

The most profound early effect is on the central nervous system, where it acts as a sedative, producing relaxation and a sense of well-being. Alcohol is sometimes used as an antidepressant for people who try to self-diagnose themselves. It impairs the intellect, physical abilities, and metabolism. When alcohol is taken regularly in large amounts over many years, permanent physical damage will occur. This damage is often aggravated by the lack of vitamins because most alcoholics have poor eating habits. Alcohol can also damage the liver, brain, and other parts of the nervous system. In the final stages of alcoholism, parts of the brain are permanently damaged and confusion, disorientation, and delirium tremens (DTs) result.

Alcohol changes brain cells, impairs physical coordination, causes memory loss, and irritates the stomach lining, causing gastrointestinal problems. Heavy drinking can lead to high blood pressure, and irregular heart rhythms, and it increases the chances of heart failure and stroke. The liver is especially compromised since it filters alcohol out of the body. Chronic drinking causes cirrhosis of the liver. Alcohol is destructive to the immune system by inhibiting white blood cells from fighting infection, thereby, increasing the risk of viral or bacterial infections and cancers.

Deep inside the brain, alcohol can affect the areas that control aggression, hunger and thirst, pleasure and pain, and body temperature. These effects are produced because alcohol inhibits blood from transporting oxygen to brain cells. When brain cells are deprived of oxygen, they become impaired and die. The hypothalamus is the portion of the brain that controls automatic reflexes: breathing, heartbeat, and other bodily operations over which an individual has no conscious control. When alcohol is present in the bloodstream, it directly affects the hypothalamus, possibly damaging it, particularly during the adolescent years. In addition, alcohol has a profound effect on the frontal lobe, the part of the brain that allows us to analyze and program our behavior. It also allows us to convert experience to memory and is responsible for the formation of our self-image. These processes require a tremendous amount of energy. The depressant nature of alcohol and other toxic chemicals directly lowers the energy center in the brain, resulting in the loss not only of mental capacity but the ability to realize that it is lost and judgment is impaired.

The disinhibiting effect of alcohol is one of the main reasons it is used in so many social situations. Alcohol is a drug that produces dual effects on the body. The first is a primary depressant effect that lasts a short time, then a secondary central nervous system effect kicks in that lasts six times longer. In a quiet, nonsocial setting, the drug may inhibit any excitatory transmission, resulting in sedation and drowsiness. In a social setting, the drug may enhance excitement (disinhibition) such as talkativeness, increased self-confidence, and general loss of self-restraint. As doses increase, so do the behaviors of slurred speech, staggering, loss of emotional control, severe respiratory depression, coma, and death. Hangovers are an after-effect of consumption of alcohol, consisting of headaches, nausea, thirst, dizziness, and fatigue.

Fetal alcohol syndrome is the most serious condition associated with drinking during pregnancy. Alcohol has teratogenic effects which can result in birth defects and mental retardation. They are characterized by low birth weight, small head, and failure to thrive and grow properly. Neurological deficits include poor coordination and sleep patterns, jitteriness, learning disabilities, hyperactivity, short attention span, and behavioral difficulties. The striking feature is craniofacial malformations, an irreversible physical abnormality. Women who drink during their pregnancies double the risk of having a baby born with physical or mental deficits.

Infants born to alcoholic mothers may be born addicted and may experience withdrawal symptoms at birth. A recent study has found that a father's drinking habits during the month of his child's conception can affect his baby's birth weight. Most of these are problems that will last a lifetime.

"Due to my drinking, I lost his bed at the Rescue Mission and began sleeping down in the bushes by the Missouri River. One morning, I woke up and there were rats crawling all over me. I grabbed a rock and tried to smash them, but I couldn't hit any of them. That's when I knew they were all in my mind. It was the DT's again." (Eric Newhouse 2001)

Alcoholism is defined as a "chronic, progressive, and potentially fatal disease marked by repeated drinking that causes trouble in the drinker's personal, professional, and family life." (The National Council on Alcoholism) World Health Organization reports that 2.5 million people die from this disease every year. In the United States, about 18 million people have an alcohol-use disorder known as dependence, alcoholism, or alcohol abuse. Alcoholism is a disorder or disease with symptoms and signs that may include the following:

- Craving—a persistent need or urge to drink.
- Loss of control—not being able to stop drinking once intoxicated.
- Chronic disease—in which a person spends a great deal of time drinking or recovering from its effects.
- Physical dependence—withdrawal symptoms and physical need for alcohol.
- Tolerance—the need to drink greater amounts to feel good or normal.
- Withdrawal—body and mind require alcohol to remain stable, otherwise a person may experience anxiety, psychosis, and, in extreme cases, death.
- Efforts to quit—a person may abandon life's major functions such as work, marriage, and children because the drug has become too important. He or she may try to quit and relapse back to the behavior.

Early alcoholic drinking may produce the following specific medical conditions:

- Loss of control of eye muscles
- Hypoglycemia
- Gastritis
- Increased susceptibility to infections
- Cardiac arrhythmia
- Anemia
- Constant flushing of face; facial edema

- Peripheral neuritis
- Pancreatitis
- Increase in blood alcohol level
- Withdrawal signs
- Fatty liver
- Increase in blood pressure

Chronic alcohol drinking produces even more severe conditions, some of which may be irreversible, such as:

- Liver damage
- Krokoff syndrome (Vitamin B deficiency)
- Brain damage
- Cardiomyopathy
- Cancer of the tongue, mouth, or pharynx, hypopharynx, esophagus, and liver

As with other addictions, such as smoking, alcohol consumption is a learned behavior—no one likes the taste of alcohol at first. People drink out of curiosity, custom, or to escape from an unpleasant feeling to gain a sense of well-being and euphoria. It is a primary disease, not caused by some underlying psychological or moral flaw; it is chronic and does not go away with time; it is progressive and does not improve as long as one continues to drink; and it is a potentially fatal disease if the drinking is not interrupted.

Four stages of drinking progression to alcoholism:

- Stage One—a person experiments with alcohol and may feel good; after the effects wear off, drinker returns to normal.
- Stage Two—a person starts socially drinking more often and may get drunk often without experiencing anything more than a hangover.
- Stage Three—a person experiences anticipation and preoccupation with drinking; becomes dependent on alcohol to make it through the day.
- Stage Four—a person becomes a full blown alcoholic; blackouts, repression, and euphoric recall are common occurrences.

In a blackout state, the alcoholic may function as if he or she is aware of what is going on, but when sober, he or she usually cannot remember the event that took place. Repression is the defense the mind uses to push events back into the subconscious because they maybe too painful; many behaviors while drinking may produce great shame or pain. Euphoric recall allows the alcoholic to remember the good parts of the drinking binge.

Characteristics of Alcohol Intoxication
Significant problematic behavior
Psychological changes
Impaired functioning and judgment
Poor coordination interfering with driving abilities
Amnesia or blackouts
Life-threatening body systems failure and coma

These are the stages of recovery an addict typically works through:

- First stage in recovery for an alcoholic begins with breaking through the denial and admitting he or she has a problem.
- Second stage is realizing how serious the condition has become and that he or she needs help.
- Third stage is acceptance and commitment in his or her recovery, taking responsibility for his or her personal health.
- Fourth stage is surrender in which the patient learns self-acceptance and begins close relationships again.

Alcohol withdrawal syndrome occurs with sudden cessation of long-term, extensive alcohol intake. Withdrawal symptoms include severe anxiety, sweating, nausea, vomiting, tremors, hallucinations, delirium tremens, and alcoholic seizures (convulsions). Long-term effects of consuming large quantities of alcohol, especially when combined with poor nutrition, can lead to permanent damage to vital organs such as the brain, heart, pancreas, and liver. An alcoholic may need to be placed in a detoxification center for supportive care to get through the withdrawal symptoms. The Kindling model of sedative hypnotic (substance) withdrawal results from repeated withdrawal occurrences. Each withdrawal leads to more severe withdrawal symptoms. This increasing severity of withdrawal symptoms includes increased risk of seizures.

The signs of alcohol withdrawal syndrome are:

- Autonomic hyperactivity: tremors, delirium, seizures, tachycardia, increased temperature
- Anxiety, confusion, headache
- Insomnia, nightmares, sweats

- Mental disturbances, delirium tremens
- Perception distortions, spinning
- Gastrointestinal symptoms, nausea, vomiting
- Significant disturbance or impairment in social, occupational, or other functioning
- Develops within several hours to a few days after cessation of or reduction in heavy, prolonged alcohol use.
- Peak intensity during second day of abstinence with improvement likely by the fourth or fifth day.
- Symptoms may continue for up to 3–6 months at lower intensity levels

The recovery is defined as meeting the diagnostic criteria for full remission of alcohol use; in other words, abstinence from alcohol. Self-help groups and Alcoholics Anonymous have become widely used around the world. Cognitive-behavior therapy, which teaches skills for coping along with common triggers for relapse, is also useful.

Treatment options for alcohol use disorder include:

- Counseling and psychological techniques and therapies
- Twelve-Step (self-help) Programs
- Cognitive-behavioral therapies (various)
- Behavioral self-control training (BSCT): teaching skills that target controlled drinking as a treatment goal
- Moderation-oriented cue exposure (MOCE): designed to train moderation of alcohol consumption
- Guided self-change (GSC): cognitive-behavioral motivational intervention to assist drinkers in recognizing and utilizing personal strengths to resolve problems
- Motivational interviewing (MI): based on the idea that motivation is a fluctuating trait which can be positively influenced to enhance the seeking of treatment

Drug options for alcohol use disorder include:

Disulfiram (Antabuse®) blocks an enzyme, acetaldehyde dehydrogenase, that metabolizes alcohol, provoking an intense physical response such as nausea, headache, palpitations, and vomiting when alcohol is ingested. This aversion therapy medication has significant adverse effects with no clear evidence of craving reduction, increased abstinence, or reduction of relapse rates. There is a high noncompliance rate.

Naltrexone (ReVia®) reduces cravings for alcohol within the brain's dopamine system. It is an opioid-receptor antagonist. By blocking opioid receptors, the high feelings of intoxication are reduced, thereby, the thinking and cravings for alcohol are dampened. The side effect profile includes nausea, headache, anxiety, and sedation. Patients who have hepatitis, liver failure, are on long-term opioid therapy for chronic pain, and those who are heroin dependent should not take naltrexone.

Acamprosate's (Campral®) mechanism is unclear, but it is useful to stabilize the brain that would otherwise be disrupted by alcohol withdrawal. The chemical structure is similar to GABA and may partially enhance the effect on GABA receptors. The drug is thought to block glutaminergic N-methyl-D-aspartate receptors, thereby, dampening alcohol's effect on the neural reward pathways while easing withdrawal symptoms. The drug is safe, well tolerated, and with minimal side effects except for transient diarrhea. Patients who have renal insufficiency and advanced cirrhosis should not take acamprosate.

Naltrexone extended release parenteral suspension (Vivitrol®) is a once monthly injection that elevates plasma naltrexone. This type of dosage form improves patient adherence and compliance to therapy.

Topiramate (Topamax®) for craving reduction is thought to work by blocking the release of the neurotransmitter dopamine. Dopamine is associated with the reward triggers and cravings.

Nalmefene (Selincro®) is an opioid receptor antagonist used in the management of alcohol dependence, which significantly reduces alcohol consumption better than placebo. Side effects: nausea, dizziness, insomnia, and headache.

Quetiapine (Seroquel ®) is an atypical antipsychotic which has shown to be more effective in increasing abstinence and reducing heavy drinking than placebo.

Baclofen (Lioresal®) has been found to suppress symptoms of alcohol withdrawal syndrome, reduce cravings, and help prevent relapse in alcohol dependence patients. It is a GABA receptor agonist.

Adjunct therapy: Benzodiazepines for short-term withdrawal management. Antidepressants for depression. Antipsychotics for hallucinations.

Cannabis

Cannabis contains the chemical compound THC or delta-9 tetrahydrocannabinol. It is used for hemp fiber, for hemp oils, for medicinal purposes, and as a recreational drug. The popularity as a recreational drug is worldwide and is ranked just below alcohol, caffeine, and tobacco. Cannabis has primary psychoactive effects such as causing a state of relaxation or euphoria. Its secondary psychoactive effects can include introspection, metacognition, anxiety, and paranoia. It can also increase heart rate and hunger. Cannabis has a lower risk factor for dependence compared to nicotine or alcohol. Its withdrawal symptoms include irritability and insomnia.

According to Deborah Malka, M.D., cannabis is the material derived from the herbaceous plant cannabis. Cannabis contains more than 400 chemicals and has many effects seen throughout the body. Cannabis has long-term effects that include mood disturbances in otherwise healthy individuals, including depression, apathy, and social isolation. Some neurological effects include increases in regional cerebral blood flow, reduction in REM sleep while increasing overall sleep, and impairment in recent memory recall. THC has an antinociceptive (analgesic) effect and can be used for pain. Exogenous cannabinoids mimic the effects of endogenous cannabinoids in the CNS by decreasing the binding of calcium ions on the neuronal presynaptic cleft. This promotes an analgesic effect.

Medical marijuana users praise cannabis's ability to help with nausea and assist with appetite in HIV and cancer patients undergoing chemo. Cannabis helps people control pain and anxiety and often eases the severity and duration of epileptic seizures. Cannabis reactions vary by individual, some exhibit euphoria and relaxation while others, depending on the strain, find it stimulating or mildly sedating and helpful with insomnia. Others find that short-term use of cannabis impairs thinking and coordination; in long-term studies, cannabis has been linked to lower IQs, addiction, heart, and lung complications, mental illness, car accidents, poor school outcomes, poor quality of life, and poor job performance.

Pharmacokinetics of cannabis follows accumulation dosing and is most potent via the pulmonary route of administration. Pipes, cigarettes, and water pipes minimize the acrid and irritating smoke. The effects of cannabis are felt within minutes and reach their peak in 10 to 30 minutes, with effects that may linger for two or three hours. Powdered hashish and marijuana are mixed with foods and ingested. Peak effect is within 4–6 hours with duration of 5–12 hours. THC is metabolized by liver with over 80 metabolites eliminated in the bile and feces. THC elimination half-life range is 10–13 days, with some metabolites lasting 50 hours to 6 days. Marijuana detection time is based on usage test periods for urine, blood, saliva, and hair up to 90–120 days. It can affect the metabolism of other drugs. THC is a highly lipid soluble and can be stored in fat cells potentially for several months. The stored THC is released very slowly,and unevenly back into the bloodstream.

THC in cannabis binds to cannabinoid receptors throughout the body, and marijuana's "high" comes from THC's binding to brain regions responsible for pleasure, time perception, and pain, according to the National Institute on Drug Abuse. The binding, in turn, triggers a chemical reaction that stimulates the production of dopamine, the brain chemical called the "feel-good" chemical, which is part of the body's reward system. The pharmacodynamics affect the two types of cannabinoid receptors (CB). CB1 in the brain is critical for neurological and psychological function (basal ganglia, cerebellum, and cerebral cortex). CB2 is found in the periphery and immune system.

THC cannabinoid system is potentially linked to memory by acting on CB1 receptors in the hippocampus, to appetite by acting on CB1 receptors in the hypothalamus, and to movement by acting on CB1 receptors in the cerebellum. THC binding to receptor causes a disruptive effect on the cell membrane, which may inhibit potassium (K+) channels and glutamate release. All cannabis acts as CNS depressant, depressing higher brain function, which releases lower centers from inhibitory influences. It is classified as a sedative hypnotic, anesthetic, or psychedelic due to its alteration of perceptions, thoughts, and feelings. As doses increase, its influences proceed from relief of anxiety, inhibition, and excitement to anesthesia, vasomotor depression, and collapse, with high doses producing anxiety reactions. Potential clinical uses include as an antiemetic and for anorexia, pain, muscle spasms, and neuroprotection.

Cannabis has pulmonary effects and can cause mild airway and bronchial irritations. The cardiovascular effect of cannabis is a mild lowering of blood pressure while its effect on the immune system comes from it having immune suppressant properties, thus, decreasing host resistance to infection. Cannabis has muscular effects as it is an anti-ataxic and may have anticonvulsant effects. The gastrointestinal effects are decreased muscle spasms of the GI tract, decrease in nausea and vomiting, and it is helpful in chemotherapy. Psychological effects of cannabis produce euphoria, relaxation and enhanced sensitivity, panic, anhedonia, dysphoric mood changes, poor judgement, and difficulty concentrating. The effects experienced by the cannabis user are variable and will depend upon the dose, method of administration, prior experience, any concurrent drug use, personal expectations, mood state, and the social environment in which the drug is used.

Effects of cannabis include:

- An altered state of consciousness.
- User may feel "high," very happy, euphoric, relaxed, sociable, and uninhibited.
- Distorted perceptions of time and space.
- User may feel more sensitive to things around him or her and may also experience a more vivid sense of taste, sight, smell, and hearing.
- Increased pulse and heart rate, bloodshot eyes, dilated pupils, and often increased appetite.
- Impaired coordination and concentration, making activities such as driving a car or operating machinery difficult and dangerous.
- Anxiousness, panic, self-consciousness, and paranoid thoughts.

CNS Systems Effect

- Mind-altering properties
- Anxiety free state, well-being
- Time and space distortions
- Ideas flow, disconnected, impaired memory, perception
- Gaps in thought similar to absence seizure
- Palpitations, light headed, floating
- Weakness, tremors, hypotension,
- Incoordination, amotivational
- Hallucinations in high doses
- Dissociative phenomena (mental processes become separate from normal consciousness)
- Subjective altered state of consciousness

People who use large quantities of cannabis may become sedated or disoriented and may experience toxic psychosis. This condition manifests as not knowing who they are, where they are, or what time it is. High doses may also cause fluctuating emotions, fragmentary thoughts, paranoia, panic attacks, hallucinations, and feelings of unreality.

Long-term effects of heavy use can include:

- Irritation to the lungs, risk of developing chronic bronchitis, and an increased risk of developing cancer of the respiratory tract (more likely to do with smoking).
- Exacerbation of preexisting cardiovascular disease as cannabis use significantly raises the heart rate.
- Decreased concentration levels, reduced short-term memory, and difficulties with thinking and learning (resolved if cannabis use stops).
- Decreased sex drive in some people. Chronic use can lower sperm count in males and lead to irregular periods in females (resolved if cannabis use stops).
- Dependence on cannabis—compulsive need to use the drug, coupled with problems associated with chronic drug use.

Serious Psychological Effects

- Fear, panic, paranoia
- Disorientation, memory loss, confusion,
- Acute psychotic reactions
- Toxic psychoses
- Long-term anxiety, schizophrenia, and depression with regular use

Drug options for cannabis use include:

Dronabinol (Marinol) is THC in sesame oil as a prophylaxis of nausea in cancer patients. It has shown to be superior to placebo. For stimulation of appetite in patients with AIDS and anorexia, with results of inconsistent weight gain. Other products include Nabilone.

(Cesamet), Delta9-THC (Sativex), and Rimonabant (Acomplia). Withdrawal symptoms include insomnia, anxiety, irritability, and restlessness which may persist for weeks. The drug craving may persist intermittently for months. Treatment is supportive care and nonpharmacologic interventions.

Contradictory information exists regarding marijuana and pregnancy. Studies have found that prenatal marijuana use can cause premature birth, low birth weight, and a higher risk of stillbirth. Marijuana use in the third trimester can lead to the child presenting with temporary withdrawal-like symptoms, increased tremors, and crying at birth. These children may have differences in brain activity, behavior, and sleeping patterns. However, evidence is not conclusive, and some studies report conflicting results. Mothers who breastfeed their children while using marijuana can pass the drug on to their children through the milk. Marijuana use may also affect the quality and quantity of the breast milk.

Tibor Harkany, a neuroscientist at the Karolinski Institute in Sweden, and the Medical University of Vienna shared a study in the EMBO Journal called "Eleven Facts Every Parent Should Know About Their Baby's Brain." The Harkany Study found that exposure to marijuana very early in life may negatively affect brain development. He stated that a concentration of THC late in pregnancy could have profound and long-lasting consequences for the brain. The data confirmed that the fetal brain, at a molecular level, is particularly sensitive to THC and that prenatal cannabis use disrupts synapses and nerve connections that are critical for cognitive function. It shared that school age children, prenatally exposed to marijuana, are more likely to show gaps in problem solving, memory, and attention span. Harkany stated, "Any drug that interferes with a child's development is detrimental to that child." Harkany concluded that to determine the real risks of marijuana use during pregnancy, more research is needed. Harkanys' warning for women is to advise pregnant mothers not use marijuana.

According to the Marijuana Cannabis Prevention Information Center, when both parents use marijuana during a pregnancy, there is a higher risk of SIDS, sudden infant death syndrome. The center reported that at the age of six months, children who were prenatally exposed to marijuana use are at a greater risk for asthma, chest infections, and other breathing problems. By age three or four, the same children are recorded to have poorer verbal skills and difficulties with memory and reasoning. Their motor skills are often delayed, and they are more likely to be fearful, impulsive, inattentive, and hyperactive. By the age of ten, children exposed to marijuana during gestation are dealing with problems that have persisted since birth. They may experience additional issues with reading and spelling, depression and anxiety, and become underachievers at school. The problems these children experience may continue through adolescence and early adulthood.

A landmark study by Melanie Dreher, RN, PHd, FAAN, a medical anthropologist, conflicts with all the other information on marijuana and pregnancy. Dreher's study in Jamaica lasted ten years and involved mothers of babies who used marijuana during pregnancy and mothers who did not. The mothers who used marijuana did so daily for morning sickness or nausea, to prevent depression and fatigue, and to improve their appetites. Dreher concluded that there was no difference in birth weight or the neuro tests given to the babies at birth. Testing these same children at the 30-day mark showed that the children of the mothers that smoked marijuana had a better organization of sleeping and waking and were prone to less stress-related anxiety.

She reported that the babies of the marijuana-using mothers made eye contact more quickly, socialized more quickly, were easier to engage than the other babies, and had better self-regulation. Dreher reported no signs of birth defects or behavioral problems in marijuana-exposed children during their first months or after several years. The study showed that after five years of studying both groups, nothing linked to the babies' development was due to exposure to marijuana. After spending 30 years researching marijuana use during pregnancy Melanie Dreher indicted that there are lots of studies that have gone unpublished that would lend support to a very different picture of prenatal cannabis exposure.

Hypnotics

The term hypnotic encompasses medications and therapeutic classifications that include antianxiety agents used in the treatment of anxiety, panic disorders, and sleep disorders. They affect primary motor skills and thought, central nervous system neurotransmitters, acetylcholine (Ach), aspartate, dopamine, norepinephrine, serotonin, GABA (inhibitory), and glutamate (excitatory).

Cumulative stress is dependent upon our individual reframing of perception, learning coping skills, and self-care. Symptoms of stress, anxiety, and panic include high sensitivities of uneasiness, worry, apprehension, and fearful feelings as a response that interferes with quality of life.

Sleep disorders can be categorizes as transient, resulting from stress or change, lasting a few days in duration; short term, resulting from a persistent major life stressor, lasting up to three weeks in duration; chronic, resulting from a medical or psychological illness.

Sleep and Relaxation Hygiene

Arise same time
Avoid daytime naps
Avoid alcohol, large meals, nicotine, caffeine
Set up a good sleep area
Increase exercise
Meditation, breathing
Drink warm milk (natural source of tryptophan)
Use alternative medicines (Valerian Root, Melatonin)
OTC antihistamines (Diphenhydramine, Doxylamine)

Barbiturates

Barbiturates have seen a decline in use and are no longer utilized as the drug of choice due to high addiction potential, adverse effects, slow onset, low therapeutic index, and availability of more effective agents. They have narrow therapeutic ranges with a high potential for lethal overdose, tolerance, dependence, abuse, and dangerous drug interactions. The pharmacokinetics of oral barbiturate dosing is sedation within 20–30 minutes, with a residual hangover effect. The agent is eliminated via the kidneys. Common names are phenobarbital, pentobarbital, yellow jackets, secobarbital, red devils, amobarbital, and blue devils. Barbiturates' mechanism of action and pharmacodynamics activity include:

- Depression of neuronal pathways in brain stem and cerebral cortex
- Reduction of electrical and metabolic brain activity
- Increase of dosage that causes deep coma, cessation of respiration, and death
- Barbiturates that bind to GABA receptors, the inhibitory neurotransmitter

Barbiturates' Central Nervous System Depressants' Effects

- Depressed blood pressure and respiration
- Drowsiness, constricted pupils
- Impaired judgment
- Slurred speech, confusion
- Depressed tendon reflexes
- Coma, shock, confusion

Barbiturates are distributed to the fetus. Data suggest developmental abnormalities can occur.

Barbiturates need to be avoided during pregnancy. A risk versus benefit analysis is recommended to change to another antiepileptic agent if warranted.

Benzodiazepines

Benzodiazepines have many therapeutic roles and are typically well tolerated in the general population. Benzodiazepines are one of the most widely prescribed pharmacologic agents in the United States. They are used for numerous indications, including anxiety, insomnia, muscle relation, relief from spasticity caused by central nervous system pathology, and epilepsy.

These drugs are also used because of their amnesic and anxiolytic properties. The exact mechanism of action of benzodiazepines is not fully known. They appear to work in the brain by enhancing the effects of gamma-aminobutric acid (GABA), a brain chemical that is naturally calming. Benzodiazepines work on the GABA receptor to increase its sensitivity to inhibitor stimuli, thereby, slowing down or blocking certain nerve signals. It affects the central nervous system and is classified as a depressant.

Pharmacodynamics

GABA receptor interactions

- Three dimensional change to receptor
- Benzodiazepine agonists, eg., diazepam
- Benzodiazepine antagonists, eg., flumazenil
- Influx of chloride ion channels and depressing excitability

Local Brain Pharmacodynamics

- Low-dose antianxiety effects: hippocampus and amygdala
- Mental confusion and amnesia: hippocampus and cerebral cortex
- Sedative-hypnotic effects: cerebral cortex
- Different benzodiazepines have different relative effects, perhaps due to multiple subtypes of GABA receptors

Unfortunately, side effects and toxicity can result in morbidity and mortality in a small number of patients. The elderly, patients with lung, liver, or kidney dysfunction, and patients on other classes of medication are especially prone to toxicity. Common side effects of benzodiazepines include fatigue, confusion, dizziness, euphoria, mood swings, slurred speech, vision change, amnesia. Overdose, particularly when combined with other drugs, can lead to respiratory depression, coma, and death. Flumazenil is a benzodiazepine receptor antagonist used to treat benzodiazepine overdoses. It has a short half-life and requires multiple intravenous doses and patient monitoring.

The severity of benzodiazepines-induced adverse effects has cautioned physicians to pay close attention to side effects when prescribing this class of agents. Tolerance, dependence, age-related physiological changes, and drug interactions are all important factors to take into consideration. The newer high-potency drugs in this class show improved therapeutic effects as well as foster onset of action, making them the preferred choices for most patients. However, with increased potency comes an increase in the risk of undesired effects. Therefore, when prescribing drugs in this group, physicians must consider individual properties such as absorption, distribution, elimination half-life, and lipid solubility. Benzodiazepines are not recommended for use in chronic anxiety disorders, in the elderly, for depression, for short-term treatment of stress-related anxiety—either acute situational grief or acute stress reactions—and for short-term anxiety-induced insomnia.

All benzodiazepines can cause physical dependence. If benzodiazepines are taken continuously for longer than a few months, suddenly discontinuing therapy may result in withdrawal symptoms. Symptoms may include tremors, muscle cramping, vomiting, sweating, feeling of loss of self-worth, agitation, insomnia, feeling nervous or tense, being confused or depressed, feeling afraid or paranoid, anxiety, panic, feelings of disconnection, altered sensorium, and shaking or convulsions. In order to avoid withdrawal symptoms, the dose of benzodiazepines must be slowly tapered.

There are about over 30 different benzodiazepines, differing in onset of action, duration, side effect profile, and toxicities. Long-acting BZD must be avoided in the elderly due to increased risk of falls and dementia. It is possible to become dependent on them after as little as four weeks, so use for short period of time if feasible.

Selected Benzodiazepine Therapeutic Agents

- Diazepam (Valium)
- Chlordiazepoxide (Librium)
- Alprazolam (Xanax)
- Clonazepam (Klonopin)
- Lorazepam (Ativan)
- Triazolam (Halcion)
- Clorazepate (Tranxene)
- Oxazepam (Serax)
- Temazepam (Restoril)
- Midazolam (Versed)

Benzodiazepine Pharmacokinetics

- Metabolized in the liver.
- Intermediate metabolites may be psychoactive.
- Intermediate metabolites may be long lasting.
- Elderly patients have difficulty metabolizing long-acting benzodiazepines, leading to profound dementia. May take 60 days to clear.
- ProSom, Dalmane, Restoril, Halcion primarily used for insomnia.

- Clonazepam (Klonopin) is preferred for long treatment of alcohol dependence.
- Lorazepam, Diazepam, Chlordiazepoxide (Librium) are favored for short-term, acute treatment of alcohol withdrawal.

Drug options for benzodiazepine use include:
Alprazolam is a short-acting high potency drug with an elimination half-life of 6–27 hours. This drug is used for panic disorders and is proven to be well tolerated and effective. A common issue with alprazolam is rebound anxiety that occurs with abrupt discontinuation because of the drug's short elimination half-life.

Lorazepam is another high potency drug that displays short-acting characteristics. It is a slightly less lipid soluble compared with alprazolam, suggesting a lower risk of amnesic side effects compared to alprazolam. Lorazepam has proven effective as an anticonvulsant and also works well as an adjunct to antipsychotics in the treatment of acute agitation and mania. Following intramuscular injection, lorazepam is absorbed rapidly and completely. After sublingual administration, lorazepam reaches peak plasma levels in roughly 60 minutes. Lorazepam has been proven to work in patients with hepatic or renal dysfunction with only minor effects on the drug's pharmacokinetics.

Diazepam is a useful muscle relaxer and a treatment for status epilepticus and alcohol withdrawal. It is unique in that its metabolism in the liver produces the active metabolites oxazepam, temazepam, and desmethydiazepam, each of which exerts its own action. These metabolites and their actions account for diazepam's long elimination half-life. The half-life increases one hour for each year of age over 40. Example: The diazepam elimination half-life in a 75-year-old would be approximately 75 hours. Physicians must take this into consideration when prescribing the drug. If they are not cautious, it is possible to cause an active metabolite buildup, such as oversedation and anterograde amnesia. These side effects can be serious and long lasting, especially in the elderly and in those with hepatic or renal dysfunction.

Diazepam is used for anxiety. It can be administered either intramuscularly or intravenously. Common side effects among benzodiazepines are drowsiness, lethargy, and fatigue. At higher dosages, impaired motor coordination, dizziness, vertigo, slurred speech, blurry vision, mood swings, and euphoria can occur, as well as hostile or erratic behavior in some instances. Tolerance, dependence, and withdrawal are adverse effects associated with long-term use. Veno-irritation may occur with diazepam and lorazepam. Both of these agents are commonly administered in a hospital or a palliative care setting in intravenous formulations.

Delirium is probably one on the worst adverse effects of benzodiazepines. This is commonly seen in the intensive care setting. Delirium is an acute condition characterized by impaired attention and cognition. Benzodiazepines increase the risk of delirium, especially in elderly patients in the intensive care unit. Delirium is a serious problem and can lead to increased morbidity, increased mortality, and longer hospital stays. Morbidity and mortality increase because the risk of nosocomial infections increases the longer the patient stays in the hospital. Physicians need to be cautious of the risks of delirium when administering these drugs to hospitalized patients.

Benzodiazepines have shown clear evidence of risk to the fetus. It is a teratogen, increasing the risk of prenatal abnormalities and birth complications. These include neural tube defect, ventricular septal defect, heart defect, CNS abnormalities, abnormally small head, wide eye sets, limb deformities, urogenital abnormalities, scalp aphasia, cutis congentia, retarded fetal growth, skull defect, craniofacial defects, underdeveloped jaw, and oral clefts. The likelihood and severity of the defects may be affected by the level of exposure and the stage of pregnancy in which it occurred. Early reports suggested that there may be an increased risk of cleft lip and palate associated with first trimester exposure to these medications, estimating the risk to be about 0.7%; however, more recent studies have suggested that the risk may be even lower. Since this risk is restricted to the first trimester, a risk versus benefit analysis may be used to determine overall risk of teratogenesis during the second and third trimesters. Benzodiazepines use in pregnancy can cause toxicity and withdrawal symptoms in the infant, sucking difficulties, irritability, sleep disruption, poor muscle tone or floppiness (floppy infant syndrome), poor temperature control, and, less commonly, seizure.

Newer agents have been developed in the non-benzodiazepine (BZRA) classification. These include zolpidem (Ambien), zaleplon (Sonata), and eszopiclone (Lunesta), which are not benzodiazepines yet act as a specific agonist at GABAA1 receptors. Rapid onset, short elimination half-life, and less risk of tolerance,and abuse make these agents an effective insomnia treatment. They show little interference with normal sleep cycle. They appear to be safe; however, high doses trigger vomiting. High doses also produce problems in older people. Flumazenil antagonizes zolpidem.

Ramelteon (Rozerem) has a high melatonin affinity as a melatonin receptor agonist. It works by fooling the body into thinking it has more melatonin, a hormone that promotes sleep. It is effective in the treatment of insomnia and has not been shown to produce any dependence, potential for abuse, withdrawal, or rebound insomnia. Buspirone (BuSpar) is a weak serotonin receptor agonist, so there is no crossing or synergy with other CNS depressants. Buspirone is also an antidepressant with no sedation and little amnesia or confusion. It has a very slow onset in about 3–4 weeks with minimal abuse and withdrawal symptoms. This agent is useful for GAD and anxiety in older people. Trazodone (Desyrel) is a serotonin antagonist and reuptake inhibitor (SARI) class that is commonly used in the treatment of both depression and insomnia. This dual activity combined with low cost and low abuse potential makes it an attractive alternative.

Gamma-Hydroxybutyrate (GHB)

GHB is an analog metabolite of the inhibitory neurotransmitter GABA. It is synthesized in the brain in small amounts and is thought to function as a neurotransmitter and neuromodulator that may be coreleased with GABA at some synapses. GHB was developed pharmacologically as a CNS-depressant compound. It was later marketed in the United States as a bodybuilding supplement until over-the-counter sales were banned in 1990. Nevertheless, illicit GHB continues to be used recreationally and, occasionally, as a date rape drug at clubs.

Another date rape drug is Rohypnol, a potent benzodiazepine. It is manufactured in Europe and illegally smuggled in or synthesized in illicit drug factories. Legal manufacturers have made changes to decrease the possibility of being placed in a drink undetected. Now, Rohypnol dissolves more slowly, turns pale drinks bright blue and dark drinks murky, and contains insoluble particles that float to the top of the glass.

GHB is usually taken orally in the form of an aqueous solution. Low doses produce alcohol-like effects, including mild euphoria, relaxation, and social disinhibition. Higher doses are associated with stronger sedating effects as well as dizziness, nausea, vomiting, and memory impairment. Severe overdosing with GHB causes severe respiratory depression, unconsciousness, and even coma. Animals treated with GHB exhibit sedation, reduced locomotors activity, decreased anxiety behavior, and catalepsy at high doses. Impaired spatial learning has also been reported, which may be related to neurotoxic effects on the hippocampus. High doses of GHB can lead to EEG excitation, resembling absence (petit mal) seizures in humans.

The literature on GHB reinforcement is inconsistent; however, there is evidence that the drug has rewarding and reinforcing properties under the right experimental conditions. The functional effects of GHB are mediated by multiple mechanisms. The low levels of endogenous GHB are believed to act on putative high-affinity GBH-specific receptors and, possibly, also on GABA receptors. High levels of exogenously administered GHB are additionally capable of activating GABA receptors, which mediate many of the behavioral and physiological effects observed in GHB-treated animals. The sodium salt of GHB (also called sodium oxybate, trade name Xyrem) is approved in the United States for the treatment of the sleep disorder, narcolepsy. This treatment improves nighttime sleep and reduces the incidence of daytime sleepiness and attacks of catalepsy. Under the trade name Alcover, sodium oxybate is approved in Italy and Austria for the treatment of alcoholism.

Recreational GHB users reportedly experience euphoria, heightened sexuality, and feelings of relaxation during drug intoxication. In several respects, GHB intoxication resembles the state of alcohol intoxication, including impairment of psychomotor function and even loss of consciousness with overdose. The comedown following GHB use is characterized by sluggishness, mental confusion and amnesia, weakness, and increased arousal. Repeated GHB use can lead to tolerance, dependence, and withdrawal. Consumption patterns may escalate to dosing every two to four hours around-the-clock.

Inhalants

Inhalants are abused substances that are often obtained from everyday household items that produce CNS depression. In some cases, they trigger excitability. These substances contain volatile liquids or gases at room temperature; are used by sniffing, inhaling, or spraying the substance; and do not belong to another defined class of abused drugs. Inhalants are most commonly used by children and adolescents, and they are often the first substance of abuse tried by a child. Low doses of volatile and gaseous inhalants produce effects resembling those seen with alcohol intoxication. Users exposed to greater amounts of these substances show stronger depressant effects, including slurred speech, poor coordination, ataxia, and sleepiness. At very high doses, loss of consciousness, sensory distortions, hallucinations, and coma can occur. Repeated inhalant use can lead to tolerance, dependence, and an abstinence syndrome when drug use is stopped. Withdrawal symptoms include nausea, fatigue, irritability, anxiety, sleep disturbances, and craving.

Inhalants show reward and reinforcing properties; increased firing of DA neurons in the VTA may play a role in inhalant reward and reinforcement. Inhalants are rapidly absorbed from the lungs and quickly enter the brain from the bloodstream because of their high lipid solubility. Distribution within the brain does not appear to be uniform, and this may influence the behavioral effects of these substances. The depressant effects of inhalants, particularly toluene (which is the best studied inhalant), can generally be attributed to enhancement of inhibitory GABA receptor activity as well as to inhibition of excitatory NMDA and nicotinic receptors.

Pharmacokinetics

- Administration—sniffed
- Rapid CNS absorption from lung to bloodstream—rush < 1 minute
- Rapid CNS depression and vasodilation
- Dropped blood pressure, heart rate, oxygen consumption
- Marked inebriation, dizziness, floating sensations, exhilaration, intense feeling of well being

Pharmacodynamics

- Enhances inhibitory function on GABA
- Inhibits the excitatory NMDA glutamate receptors
- Reduces CNS excitation
- Causes behavioral impairment similar to alcohol

Inhalants present serious health risks including damage to the liver, kidneys, lungs, bone, and brain. Solvent abusers show cognitive impairment that may be related to the injurious effects of inhalants on the brain, such as white-matter abnormalities seen on MRI scans. Inhalant use can additionally lead to a rare disorder called sudden sniffing death syndrome, which in some cases results from an inhalant-induced cardiac arrhythmia. Moreover, some offspring exposed to inhalants in utero reportedly suffer from fetal solvent syndrome, which involves craniofacial abnormalities and, possibly, also cognitive deficits. These effects resemble those seen in individuals diagnosed with fetal alcohol syndrome.

Inhalant Products

- Aerosols
- Hairspray
- Vegetable Oil
- Spray Paint
- Gases, Glues
- Lighters

- Appliances
- Nitrous Oxide

Nitrates (Poppers)

- Butyl nitrite
- Now illegal
- Sold as room deodorizer
- Video head cleaners
- Leather cleaners
- Mail order
- Drug shops
- Adult bookstores

Symptoms at High Doses

- Slurred speech
- Sensory distortion
- Hallucinations
- Bronchial and laryngeal irritations
- Confusion
- Coma
- Blood dyscrasia
- Depression

Chronic Inhalant Use

- Tolerance
- Hepatic and renal toxicity
- Death from cardiac dysrhythmia
- Respiratory failure

Alpha Omega

Case #1

"I am a 44-year-old man who was living the so-called American dream. I had a home, cars, family, and a great paying job. I lost it all due to drinking. I had been drinking since the age of 12. I thought I had it all under control. I paid my bills; my wife and kids never wanted for anything. I never drank during my work week, but from the time my weekend started, I pretty much had a drink in my hand. My marriage was falling apart, and I didn't know how to cope, and I drank even more. I went from half a bottle to a whole bottle and chasing it with beer.

"One night, I had a blackout and did the unthinkable and hurt one of my kids. My wife told me what I did, and I tried to kill myself. People think I tried to kill myself out of guilt of what I did, but the truth is that I don't remember any of it and still can't believe it happened. The reason I tried to kill myself was because if anyone would hurt one of my kids, I would have hurt them, so now that I did it, I had to go. I also wanted to stop all the pain and hate I had for myself. I ended up in jail. I had never been in trouble before except for kid stuff. Now I went from working in a jail to being in jail.

"I am a veteran, and the Veterans Administration came to my rescue by finding a place of recovery services. I will never forget the day I arrived as those of us who have been clients refer to it. I was scared, I didn't know what to expect. I went from being isolated in jail to a six-man room with people I didn't know. I made it through the first night and had to start my program. I remember my first group and heard some of these stories. I thought I'm not like them, I don't need to be here. I was wrong.

"The program specifically helped me figure out when I started using alcohol as a tool to not deal with my feelings and to love myself enough to not use alcohol. We call it being present. I also learned that being of service to others is the best cure to any addiction issue. I learned so much about having a higher power when times get rough. The relationships I created with the staff are priceless because they saved my life and helped me to be present in my children's life. I have a 13-year-old son, and he said to me, 'Dad, I didn't care when you drank, but I like you better when you don't.' I cried when he said that to me." —Anonymous

Case #2

"My brother and I were very close. He was extremely social and bright. He started drinking at the age of 11. The rest of the family didn't realize he had a problem with drinking until he graduated from college and got a job as an accountant. He either blacked out or didn't show up. His friends thought he was the life of the party. Little did they know he was transitioning from a functional to a dysfunctional alcoholic. Starting at the age of 25, my brother began to rotate through various rehab programs and SLE's (Sober Living Environment). He was able to maintain a job for a while but ended up on SSDI (Social Security Disability Insurance) because of his addiction and diagnosis by a psychiatrist. My brother lived until he was 39, and then his organs shut down, and he died. My mom and I finally realized my brother was the only one who could get and stay sober. My mom and I had tried for years to help him. He was, however, my best friend growing up, and I miss him terribly." —Anonymous

Case #3

"I went to my first AA meeting when I was around seven years old. My Mom was an alcoholic and also suffered from bipolar disorder. Back in those days, they were just starting to diagnose individuals with dual diagnoses. We really were not sure what was wrong with her but had a feeling it had something to do with alcohol. I was seven and my brother was nine at the time. We called the AA hotline after finding my Mom passed out. AA actually sent a nice couple up to our house to check on her, thus, started my Mom's journey into AA and my initial exposure to the rooms. Back then, people used to smoke in meetings; I hated all the smoke, but loved the donuts! I went to lots of meetings with my Mom. I liked that I saw my Mom getting better and loved hearing THE SERENITY PRAYER and THE Promises. I can still remember this one older fella sharing, and he gave me the feeling that everything was going to be ok! HOW IT WORKS and THE STEPS confused me, being only around seven years old. It's kind of funny because The Steps and How It Works eluded me for many years until much more recently. I was really able to tell you a lot about HOW IT DOESN'T WORK!"

Case #4

"Alcohol and drugs have always been a part of my story. Today, I have one daughter and two beautiful granddaughters, six and six months. My family has struggled with trying to control the booze through the years. My Mom was able to stay sober for over 15 years. When she did go back to drinking, it came after her quickly, and she never was able to get sober again. I tried many years and many times, but she really wanted to drink more than she wanted to be sober! During a ten-year stretch when she was really suffering, I had worked my way into my own bottom and eventually started my recovery process. I stayed clean for over ten years myself, but when it came back at me, I had no tools to help keep me sober. I lost my father (health issues) and some close friends along the way. Eventually, I picked up that first drink and another severe bottom waited for me, eight years down the line here and now.

"Amazingly enough, AA was still going strong!!! Of course it was. The people who have gotten sober and stayed sober are the ones who have WORKED the PROGRAM. Today, things in my life are really, really different. I have finally been able to open myself up and really heal myself through the process of Working the 12 Steps and continuing to Work them on a daily basis. My life is full again, and I feel so grateful and blessed. I have a new wife, I'm back in school at age 55, and I'm very involved in service on a personal level as well as a Fellowship level. I have new goals and a completely different attitude and outlook on life. I have an incredible sober support system and new network of friends in recovery. Those STEPS that eluded me for so many years are now easily shared. The most wonderful things are happening in my life."

Case #5

"When I bottomed out three years ago, I was only with my first granddaughter. It was a very similar situation when I found my own Mom bottomed out. My granddaughter, who was only three and a half at the time, came into the bathroom and snuggled me. She rubbed the back of my head and asked me what was wrong. My journey up and out started right there in that moment. I opened my Heart to her and was Honest. She was the only one here, and it just started coming out!!! She was amazing and hugged me even tighter. As she left the bathroom, she stopped, leaned back in, and said, 'Grandpa, it's going to be ok, just DON'T DRINK ANYMORE' Wow, I'm crying again. I have not picked up a drink since that night, and as it turns out, that day was my Mom's birthday. She shared her Message with me after all! The next morning my life changed, and it all started by simply walking back into THE ROOMS!!!!! I have come to Believe and I'm eternally Grateful."—Anonymous

Critical Thinking

"I'm 61, disabled, and have a very low income. In general, I'm a happy and cheerful person, full of life, laughter, and love. I rent a room in a house with two other people, a man and a woman, and two dogs. I haven't lived with a dog for many years, and it's kind of fun. I've spent most of my adult life living alone and unattached. In November, I became homeless. Like many homeless people, I never thought this could happen to me. Everything was fine until a few months previous when I broke my arm and wasn't able to find a job and my funds ran out. My disability check isn't enough to pay for a place to live, utilities, and food. I am one of the fortunate ones who found a bed in a local shelter.

"Living in a shelter with 9–12 other people was the first time I have lived in a group situation, and it took some time to become adjusted. Sleeping in a room with 2–3 others, hearing their breathing (and snoring!), having very little space for belongings (just the basics) is new for me. I learned to live with very little. We all had daily chores, morning or evening, sometimes both. We had to be out of the house from 8:30 a.m. to 5:00 p.m. (4:00 p.m. in the winter months). That was, perhaps, the hardest part of being homeless. Where does one go? I usually spent my time at the library or the senior center. I was able to hook up my computer to the Internet to look for a job and cheap places to live. I parked at the library and slept in my car for several hours when I was very tired or in a lot of pain.

"I've learned that homelessness is an economic situation, not a character flaw. Since becoming homeless, I met many other homeless people and have found that homeless people are just like me and YOU. I want to dedicate the rest of my life to helping homeless and underserved people. From life experience, volunteering, and education, I possess many of the necessary skills and qualities to find a job in this area—active listening skills, compassion, resourcefulness, and helping people find their own way. However, I lack the formal education necessary to find employment in human services advocacy. That's why I've enrolled in the Human Services Drug & Alcohol Advocacy Program at college. I completed the first course in my education plan and got an A. I really enjoyed the class and am looking forward to more classes.

"My time at the shelter was up in late May, and I spent several weeks couch surfing—trying to set up a place to sleep for a night or two in advance when I could. I'm happy to share that I'm no longer homeless. After saving money during the six months I was in the shelter, I found an affordable room to rent in a shared house, and it includes utilities and Wi-Fi. I've become friends with one of my housemates, and we support each other in our endeavors. In addition to classes and studying, if I can manage it, I also hope to find time to volunteer with agencies and organizations that aid the homeless and underserved. I set myself up on gofundme.com to raise money for books, fees, etc., that are not covered by the waivers. I'm very grateful to have that waiver. So far, I've gotten enough donations to cover books. I will continue to try to raise funds from friends and family for the remaining semesters." —Anonymous

WISH

ALCOHOL

Alcohol and the Brain:

https://www.youtube.com/watch?v=zXjANz9r5Fo

How much alcohol can a pregnant woman drink:

https://www.youtube.com/watch?v=7d8jYrlOuz8

Alcohol Dementia:

https://www.youtube.com/watch?v=OdMaPmLPj-s

CANNABIS

Institute of Medical Science, Faculty of Medicine, University of Toronto: Pharmacology of Cannabinoids:

https://www.youtube.com/watch?v=jznQfMj9RWM

Brain on Marijuana:

https://www.youtube.com/watch?v=oeF6rFN9org

Cannabis and the Body:

https://youtu.be/_YCzE8SOO_g

Charlotte's Story: THC and her seizures:

https://www.youtube.com/watch?v=k-2pfwCT7So

HYPNOTICS

Pharmacology of Sedative Hypnotics and GABA Receptor:

https://www.youtube.com/watch?v=-eBUJ-1vcjk

Sedative Hypnotics: Molecules that Make You Sleep

http://thebrain.mcgill.ca/flash/a/a_11/a_11_m/a_11_m_cyc/a_11_m_cyc.html

Psychoactive Drugs: Depressants and Opioids:

https://www.youtube.com/watch?v=dOlkogaWF3M

BENZODIAZEPINES

Pharmacology of Benzodiazepines:

https://www.youtube.com/watch?v=DljXO8FuUKI

GABA, Neurotransmitters, Anxiety, and the Dangers of Benzodiazepines:

https://www.youtube.com/watch?v=8TSUS8IF8Hw

Anxiety:

http://thebrain.mcgill.ca/flash/a/a_08/a_08_p/a_08_p_anx/a_08_p_anx.html

GHB

GHB:

https://www.youtube.com/watch?v=brPf7X-Gmy8

Street GHB:

https://www.youtube.com/watch?v=MbCwxzvVgUA

INHALANTS

Effects of Inhalants:

https://www.youtube.com/watch?v=P16bcKzLgNo

Teens and Inhalant Abuse:

https://www.youtube.com/watch?v=8LpFqVyx62o

My Strange Addiction Huffing Gasoline:

https://www.youtube.com/watch?v=ib5p7F0kRWU

Drug Sandbox

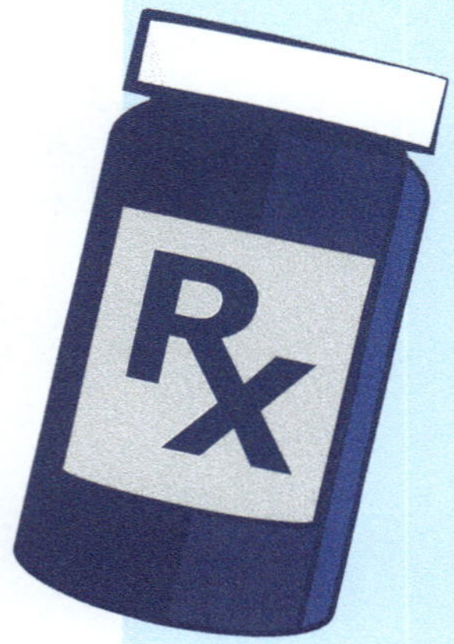

IMPORTANT WORDS TO KNOW!

Use the Internet to look up the following definitions:

Systemic Effect
Local Effect
Pharmacokinetics of Ethanol
Rate Limiting Factor
Alcohol Dehydrogenase Enzyme
Cytochrome P450
Pharmacodynamics of Ethanol
Glutamate-Nmda Receptor
Hypothalamus
Disinhibiting Effect
Dual Effects
Hangover
Fetal Alcohol Syndrome
Teratogenic Effects
Craniofacial Malformations
Alcoholism
Blackout
Stages of Recovery
Alcohol Withdrawal Syndrome
Detoxification
Kindling Model
Recovery
Disulfiram (Antabuse®)
Aversion Therapy
Naltrexone (Revia®)
Acamprosate (Campral®)

Naltrexone Extended Release Parenteral Suspension (Vivitrol®)
Topiramate (Topamax®)
Nalmefene (Selincro®)
Quetiapine (Seroquel®)
Baclofen (Lioresal®)
Adjunct Therapy
Benzodiazepines
Antidepressants
Antipsychotics
THC
Antinociceptive
Anti-Ataxic
Amotivational
Dissociative Phenomena
Toxic Psychosis
Dronabinol (Marinol®)
Nabilone (Cesamet®)
Delta9-THC (Sativex®)
Rimonabant (Acomplia®)
Hypnotic
Transient
Short Term
Chronic
Barbiturates
Narrow Therapeutic Ranges
Phenobarbital
Pentobarbital
Secobarbital
Amobarbital
Flumazenil
Alprazolam
Lorazepam
Diazepam
Active Metabolites
Oxazepam
Temazepam
Desmethydiazepam
Anterograde Amnesia
Delirium
Teratogenesis
Floppy Infant
Non-Benzodiazepine (BzRA)
Zolpidem (Ambien®)
Zaleplon (Sonata®)
Eszopiclone (Lunesta®)
Ramelteon (Rozerem®)
Buspirone (BuSpar®)
Trazodone (Desyrel®)
General Anesthetic Dissociation,
Rhabdomyolysis
Date Rape Drug
Rohypnol
Volatile Liquids or Gases
Sudden Sniffing Death Syndrome
Fetal Solvent Syndrome

Community Connections

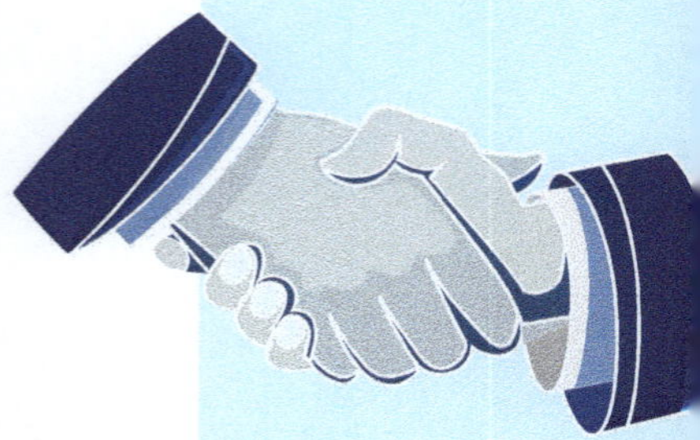

ALCOHOLIC ANONYMOUS—ONE DAY AT A TIME: IT WORKS IF YOU WORK IT

The 12-Steps Preamble states that "Alcoholics Anonymous is a fellowship of men and women who share their experience, strength, and hope with each other that they may solve their common problem and help others to recover from alcoholism. The only requirement for membership is a desire to stop drinking. There are no dues or fees for AA membership: we are self-supporting through our own contributions. AA is not allied with any sect, denomination, politics, organization, or institution: does not wish to engage in any controversy, neither endorses nor opposes any causes. Our primary purpose is to stay sober and help other alcoholics to achieve sobriety" (Grapevine).

The 12-Step Program is one that is designed especially to help an individual overcome an addiction, compulsion, serious shortcoming, or traumatic experience by emphasizing personal growth and dependence on a higher spiritual being. A 12-Step Program is a set of guiding principles, outlining a course of action for tackling problems, including alcoholism, drug addiction, and compulsion. The original 12 Steps were first published in the 1939 book Alcoholics Anonymous: The Story of How More Than One Hundred Men Have Recovered from Alcoholism. The method was adapted and became the foundation of other 12-Step Programs.

The 12 Steps Are:

1. We admitted we were powerless over alcohol—that our lives had become unmanageable.
2. Came to believe that a Power greater than ourselves could restore us to sanity.
3. Made a decision to turn our will and our lives over to the care of God as we understood Him.
4. Made a searching and fearless moral inventory of ourselves.
5. Admitted to God, to ourselves, and to another human being the exact nature of our wrongs.
6. Were entirely ready to have God remove all these defects of character.
7. Humbly asked Him to remove our shortcomings.

8. Made a list of all persons we had harmed, and became willing to make amends to them all.
9. Made direct amends to such people wherever possible, except when to do so would injure them or others.
10. Continued to take personal inventory, and when we were wrong promptly admitted it.
11. Sought through prayer and meditation to improve our conscious contact with God, as we understood Him, praying only for knowledge of His will for us and the power to carry that out.
12. Having had a spiritual awakening as the result of these Steps, we tried to carry this message to alcoholics, and to practice these principles in all our affairs.

The first three steps are taken by the individual. The alcoholic faces the truth that alcohol has gotten the best of him, that he is powerless in its grip, and that he needs help to get out of this predicament. The alcoholic at this point surrenders his will to God "or a power greater than himself" that can restore him back to sanity.

The fourth and fifth steps recommend that the alcoholic make a "searching and fearless moral inventory" of himself. He tries to see where he went wrong and how he can make things right. In the fifth step, this information is shared, usually with his sponsor. In doing this difficult step, the alcoholic finds that he is not alone in his experiences and some of the things he has done.

In the sixth and seventh steps, the alcoholic asks God (or his higher power) to remove his defects of character identified by himself and his sponsor. In steps eight and nine, the alcoholic is advised to make a list of the people he has harmed during his drinking days. This usually involves family members, loved ones, employers, employees. Self-interest is the primary motivating factor for doing these steps although it can be an embarrassing and painful process. Making amends for the wrongs you have done is a weight off your shoulders and a burden lifted from a guilty conscience.

Steps ten through twelve are referred to as maintenance steps. The alcoholic must continue to monitor his character defects, pray and meditate for guidance from his Higher Power, and, very importantly, carry the message through service and helping the newcomer, giving back what was freely given him.

The twelfth step, carrying the message of Alcoholics Anonymous, is the basic service that the AA Fellowship gives. It is the principal aim and the main reason for its existence. AA is a society of alcoholics in action. They must carry the message or else they themselves can wither, and those who have not been given the truth may die. AA service is anything that helps its members to reach a fellow sufferer, ranging from the twelfth step itself, to a phone call and a cup of coffee, to AA's General Service Office for national and international actions.

Overview: Alcoholics Anonymous is a volunteer self-help program that has no guarantees of sobriety. The fellowship uses the 12 Steps to foster a sense of belonging. The program uses suggestions rather than having standard requirements. Through time, the courts have come to use AA as a get-well setting for people struggling with alcohol and alcohol-related consequences. The AA philosophy is shared in meetings, which includes the reading of the 12 Steps. This reading starts with the word "Rarely," which goes on to suggest that if you follow the Steps, you can recover from alcoholism and your life will become increasingly better.

AA has worked miracles for alcoholics around the world. The basic principles are honesty, open-mindedness, and a willingness to work the program as it is suggested. The guidelines AA uses are guides to progress. They suggest not drinking in between meetings, reading and working out of the Big Book, getting a sponsor to take you through the steps, getting in service in the fellowship, staying in unity, and, lastly, giving back when and where you can. Many members who have found sobriety through AA have gone on to become sponsors. Sponsors are support people who can help guide you through the Steps. Sponsors usually have some good sobriety time, depending on the situation at hand. One of the main solutions the founders came to believe was that recovery from alcoholism stems from one alcoholic helping another alcoholic.

The honest sharing of experiences and behaviors has become a phenomenon in many 12-Step Programs. The Steps provide a gateway for many addicts to go back and uncover the pains and harms caused by their addictions. The process can be amazing, and many people get sober and stay sober. Getting sober and staying sober completely changes an individual's life. If the person can remain sober, usually wellness in all three aspects of the health triangle (physical, emotional social) can be seen. The key is staying sober and learning how to live sober, happy lives. Most alcoholics have found that a return to the bottle is a return to all the misery their drinking was causing them and their families in the first place.

Positive affirmations, keywords, and sayings are used as tools; for example, "Keep Coming Back," "It Works IF You Work IT," "Do The Steps," "Live and Let Live," to name a few. The group sharing process works as a kind of group therapy session. Nobody is ever forced to share or participate on any level.

Old timers encourage newcomers to participate on whatever level they are comfortable with. There are meetings that do request that if you are intoxicated, do not actively share during the meeting. Usually these folks will be looked for after the meeting to see if they would like to talk to another person in recovery. Sharing of phone numbers, meeting schedules, AA literature, newsletters with events, and AA books for sale (or free) are also a part of the meetings.

The 12-Step Program, which originally started to help alcoholics recover, has branched out to almost every avenue of addiction, including, but not limited, to gambling, narcotics, smoking, overeating, and even sex addiction. These programs are not affiliated with AA but use the same 12-Step Model as a basis for recovery. These programs continue to grow and branch out on a global level, indicating that there is a success rate. Again, these rates are hard to track due to the anonymity of the programs and other factors, such as relapse.

The main focus is on change and positive character building. By going through the Step work, individuals can find a new freedom and a new happiness. As they move along through the process, many find that their obsession to drink has been lifted and that their lives have again become manageable. Alcohol has a way of eroding the health of the individual suffering, not only physically, but emotionally, spiritually, and socially, as well. These symptoms and phases of alcoholism are clearly outlined in the Jellinek Chart. The end chronic phase is devastating to both the alcoholic and the family. If recovery is not found, many alcoholics, unfortunately, die a lonely, miserable death.

Alcoholism has no boundaries in terms of the types of people it affects. Alcoholics come from all walks of life all around the world. The sufferings and symptoms tend to be the same for most alcoholics. Alcoholics Anonymous itself has no boundaries or limitations. The only requirement is that one has an honest desire to stop drinking and the constant reminder to place principles before personalities. It works if you work it ... work ... work ... work ... stay in the Steps.

End Of Chapter Review Questions

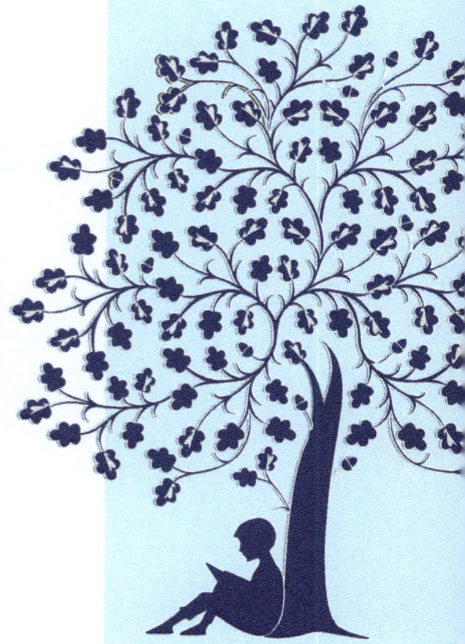

Multiple Choices: Select the best answer from the choices given:

1. Alcohol affects which of the following to the most degree?
    a. Dopamine
    b. Serotonin
    c. Glutamate-NMDA receptor
    d. Acetylcholine
    e. None of the above

2. In patients with alcohol dependence, __________ and __________ are medications that may be a benefit in maintaining abstinence from alcohol.
    a. Chloral hydrate and naltrexone
    b. Alprazolam and naltrexone
    c. Acamprosate and naltrexone
    d. Carisoprodol and naltrexone
    e. Phenobarbital and GHB

3. A program like Alcoholics Anonymous would most likely be helpful to a patient:
    a. With a history of violent behavior
    b. With high levels of anxiety
    c. With multiple additional substance addictions
    d. Without psychopathology
    e. With a lot of money

4. __________ has been associated with pregnancy-related alcohol use.
    a. Learning disabilities and behavioral problems
    b. Lipid elevation
    c. Asthma
    d. Arrhythmia
    e. None of the above

5. The rate at which the body metabolizes and eliminates alcohol is affected by:
    a. Increased body mass
    b. Reduced hepatic and renal function
    c. Sleep disturbances
    d. Cognitive decline
    e. Chronic pain

6. Which of the following are medications used in the treatment of alcohol affects alcohol dehydrogenase enzyme?
    a. Barbiturates
    b. Naloxone
    c. Alprazolam
    d. Disulfiram
    e. Acamprosate

7. __________ describes repeated withdrawal occurrences, with each withdrawal leading to more severe withdrawal symptoms.
    a. Kindling model
    b. Alcohol withdrawal syndrome
    c. Fetal alcohol syndrome
    d. Dissociative phenomena
    e. Toxic psychosis

8. __________ is THC found in sesame oil as a prophylaxis of nausea in cancer patients.
    a. Secobarbitol
    b. Dronabinol
    c. Ramelteon
    d. Gasoline
    e. Naloxone

9. __________ have seen a decline in use and are no longer utilized as the drug of choice due to addiction potential, adverse effects, and availability of more effective agents.
    a. Benzodiazepines
    b. Ethyl alcohols
    c. Ketamine
    d. GHB
    e. Barbiturates

10. __________ is a GABAA receptor antagonist used to treat benzodiazepine overdoses.
    a. Flurazepam
    b. Flumazenil
    c. Nitrous oxide
    d. Baclofen
    e. Alprazolam

11. The benzodiazepine preferred for long treatment of alcohol dependence is:
    a. Clonazepam
    b. Naloxone
    c. Ketamine
    d. Acamprosate
    e. Topiramate

12. __________is an analog of the inhibitory neurotransmitter GABA developed pharmacologically as a CNS-depressant compound.
    a. Amphetamine
    b. Nicotine
    c. Caffeine
    d. GHB
    e. Pseudoephedrine

13. __________is an opioid receptor antagonist used in the management of alcohol dependence, which significantly reduces alcohol consumption better than placebo.
    a. Phenotuatestal
    b. Flumazenil
    c. Nalmefene
    d. Buspirone
    e. Zolpidem

14. Newer agents have been developed in the nonbenzodiazepine (BZRA) classification. These include all of the following except:
    a. Zolpidem (Ambien)
    b. Zaleplon (Sonata)
    c. Eszopiclone (Lunesta)
    d. Ramelteon (Rozerem)

15. The following are methods of sleep and relaxation hygiene except:
    a. Arise same time
    b. Avoid daytime naps
    c. Avoid alcohol, large meals, nicotine, caffeine
    d. Good sleep area
    e. Stimulus before sleeping

16. Sedative hypnotics:
    a. Have a low risk of dependency
    b. Are indicated for chronic, lifetime use
    c. Affect primary motor and thought central nervous system neurotransmitters
    d. Include barbiturates, the most highly recommended drugs of choice

17. Zaleplon (Sonata) is a:
    a. Benzodiazepine hypnotic
    b. Barbiturate indicated for seizure control
    c. Nonbenzodiazepine indicated for insomnia
    d. Stimulant to treat narcolepsy

18. The following has been used in the treatment of transient insomnia:
    a. Valerian root
    b. Melatonin
    c. Diphenhydramine
    d. Doxylamine
    e. All of the above

19. __________ is unique in that its metabolism in the liver produces the active metabolites oxazepam, temazepam, and desmethydiazepam.
    a. Diazepam
    b. Pentobarbital
    c. Alprazolam
    d. Buspirone
    e. Ramelteon

20. Which of the following is a potent benzodiazepine that can be used as a date rape drug at clubs?
    a. Ramelteon
    b. Rohypnol
    c. Marinol
    d. Alprazolam
    e. Diazepam

Applications: Assessment of Usage and Relevance

1. Jill is an 89-year-old woman who has been diagnosed with an anxiety disorder.
    a. What is the pathophysiology of anxiety? Describe five physical symptoms.
    b. What medication will you recommend to the prescriber for your client? Describe the mechanism of action and rationale for your selection.
    c. Discuss pros and cons of the various anxiolytics.
    d. Discuss pros and cons of various sedative-hypnotics and their mechanism of action.
    e. What are the special considerations in this 89-year-old patient?

2. Terry is a 35-year-old Asian woman who complains of sudden episodes of shortness of breath and trembling. She feels very frightened during these episodes and feels like she is going to die. She is diagnosed with anxiety disorder.
    a. What will you recommend to the prescriber and why?
    b. What are the side effects, and how long should she expect to be on the treatment?
    c. She must attend an obligatory cocktail party. How would you advise her when she asks you, "Would it hurt if I have a cocktail or three?"
    d. What is the amnesia effect? Is Terry a candidate?
    e. Educate your client on nonpharmaceutical modalities to treat anxiety.

3. Cheyenne is a 54-year-old woman who is experiencing insomnia related to menopause. She is looking for an herbal remedy to treat insomnia temporarily until her soy products kick in.
    a. Describe the mechanism of action, efficacy, and side effects of kava.
    b. Describe the mechanism of action, efficacy, and side effects of valerian.
    c. Describe the mechanism of action, efficacy, and side effects of melatonin.
    d. What is the dosing, duration of therapy, and cost for 30 days of therapy with kava, valerian, and melatonin?
    e. How would you educate your client on nonpharmaceutical modalities to treat insomnia?

4. Edgar is a 75-year-old man who has been on Ambien 10 mg at bedtime for eight months to treat his insomnia. He presents to the emergency department and a diagnosis of overdose is made.
    a. Describe the symptoms of a benzodiazepine and nonbenzodiazepine overdose and methods of treatment.
    b. What is the mechanism of action of Ambien? What is the duration of action? Was it a good choice in this patient? Why or why not?
    c. Describe in terms of pharmacokinetics and pharmacodynamics what happened in this older adult as he increased his dosing? What can older adults experience with long-acting sedative-hypnotics?
    d. Discuss the indications and contraindications of benzodiazepines and nonbenzodiazepines and any significant drug interactions of concern.
    e. Upon discharge, Edgar indicates that the Ambien was not working anymore and that is why he took more. What is occurring? What new therapeutic agent would you suggest and why?

5. Sally, a 6-year-old girl, is taking Phenobarbital Liquid 30 mg as needed for anxiety and insomnia for three months.
    a. Describe the indications and contraindications of Phenobarbital.
    b. Describe the mechanism of action of Phenobarbital. Was this a good choice for the patient? Why or why not?
    c. List significant side effects and drug interactions of concern with Phenobarbital. What is a paradoxical reaction?
    d. What is the difference between antianxiety, sedative, and hypnotic drug effects?
    e. What special consideration is involved with children? What alternative medication would you recommend? Why?

6. The following are other agents used to treat anxiety or produce hypnosis:
    a. Summarize the drug characteristics of buspirone.
    b. Summarize the drug characteristics of hydroxyzine.
    c. Summarize the drug characteristics of chloral hydrate.
    d. Summarize the drug characteristics of ramelteon.
    e. Summarize the drug characteristics of zolpidem.

7. Outline six types of inhalants, with examples of each.

8. What are the special risks associated with inhalant abuse?

9. What are cannabinoid receptors, and where are they found? What substances act on them? What are the specific effects? In what significant brain area are they not found?

10. Explain the pharmacokinetics of marijuana and THC.

11. Explain the physiological and behavioral effects (including side effects) of marijuana use. Does it produce tolerance or dependence? Is marijuana or THC reinforcing? Evaluate the evidence.

12. Is marijuana a gateway drug? Discuss the question from at least two points of view.

13. Describe the history of use of marijuana, including the development of legal controls and their rationale.

14. Explain the categories and uses of inhalants. Who uses them and why?

KEY

1. C	6. D	11. A	16. C
2. C	7. A	12. D	17. C
3. D	8. A	13. C	18. E
4. A	9. E	14. D	19. A
5. B	10. B	15. E	20. B

REFERENCES

Alcohol

Eric Newhouse. 2001. Alcohol Cradle to Grave Center City, Minnesota Hazelden Foundation.

Janet Geringer Woititz, Ed.D. 2002. Adult Children of Alcoholics, Deerfield Beach Florida, Health Communications Inc.

George E. Vaillant. 1995. The Natural History of Alcoholism, Cambridge Massachusetts Harvard University Press.

Herma Silverstein. 1990. Alcoholism, New York, Franklin Watts, a Venture Book.

Deborah A. Dawson. 2001–2002. Recovery From Alcohol, DSM-5, pages 13–142 , nih.gov.com.

Tatiana Foround, Ph.D. 2001. Overview: Assessing the Genetic Risk for Alcohol Use Disorders, NIAAA, volume 34, issue number 3, nih.gov.

drugabuse.gov.

Cannabis

Abel, Ernest L. Effects of Prenatal Exposure to Cannabinoids. Buffalo, New York: Research Institute on Alcoholism, n.d. Print. URL, http://www.whattoexpect.com/pregnancy/marijuana/.

Hayatbakhsh, Mohammad R., et al. "Birth Outcomes Associated with Cannabis Use before and during Pregnancy." Pediatric Research 71.Number 2 (2012): 215-19. Print. Australian Study.

Healthline News, Not Stated. "Cannabis During Pregnancy Impairs Baby's Brain Development." healthline.com. Ed. Not stated. Health Line, 28 Jan. 2015. Web. 8 Sept. 2015. Online article holds position that use of marijuana during pregnancy is unsafe.

Linn, Shai, et al. "The Association of Marijuana Use with Outcome of Pregnancy." American Journal of Public Health October 1983, Vol. 73, No. 10 73.No. 10 (1983): 1161–64. Print. Scholarly review of literature in 1983.

Patients for Medical Cannibis, Not stated in blog. "Marijuana during pregnancy." Update— Dreher's research has hit mainstream media. Patients for Medical Cannibis, n.d. Web. 8 Sept. 2015. https://patients4medicalmarijuana.wordpress.com/marijuana-info/marijuana-during-pregnancy/. Quoting the author of a study in Jamaica, Dr Melanie Dreher, dean of nursing at Rush Medical Center in Chicago, published in the American Journal of Pediatrics in 1994.

Van Gelder, M. M. H. J., et al. Using Bayesian Models to Assess the Effects of Under-reporting of Cannabis Use on the Association with Birth Defects, National Birth Defects Prevention Study, 1997–2005. n.p.: n.p., 2014. Print. Pediatric and Perinatal Epidemiology 28. Abstract. URL http://www.whattoexpect.com/pregnancy/marijuana/.

What to Expect.com, Not stated. "Is It Safe to Use Marijuana during Pregnancy?" whattoexpect.com. Ed. Not provided. What to Expect.com, 22 June 2015. Web. 8 Sept. 2015. An article by an organization that provides myriad varieties of information for expectant parents. This article provides a summary of the research on the safety of marijuana use during pregnancy with links to the original sources of the information.

Wyatt, Kristen. "What Research on Pot Use during Pregnancy Does and Does Not Prove." hightimes.com. Ed. Not stated. High Times, 6 Feb. 2015. Web. 8 Sept. 2015. http://www.hightimes.com/read/what-research-pot-use-during-pregnancy-does-and-does-not-prove. Publication of an Associated Press piece. URL http://www.hightimes.com/read/what-research-pot-use-during-pregnancy-does-and-does-not-prove

University of Washington Alcohol and Drug Abuse Institute. Learn About Marijuana: Factsheets: Marijuana, Reproduction, and Pregnancy. Retrieved September 7, 2015.

CBS News http://www.cbsnews.com/news/marijuana-use-during-pregnancy-at-issue-in-colorado.

Dreher Study http://patients4medicalmarijuana.wordpress.com/marijuana-info/marijuana-during-pregnancy.

Harkany Study Karolinska Institute, Medical University of Vienna, Austria Tibor Harkany (Jan.27) in WMBO Journal "11Facts That Every Parent Should Know About Their Baby's Brain."

www.lifesciences.com/48837-marijuana.history.

O'Shaugnessy,William, On the Preparations of the Indian Hemp, or Gunjah.

Scribner, Smoke Signals: A Social History of Marijuana- edical, Recreational and Legal-(2012).

Http://adai.uw.edu/marijuana/factsheets/reproduction.htm#thash.ZLxPVsYj.dpuf.

Marijuana Cannabis Prevention and Information Center.

Http://adai.uw.edu/marijuana/factsheets/reproduction.htm#thash.ZLxPVsYj.dpuf.

NIH-National Institute on Drug Abuse.

http://www.drugabuse.gov/publications/research-reports/marijuana/can-marijuana-use-pregnancy.

http://adal.uw.edu/marijuana/factsheets/whatiscannabis.htm.

http://adai.uw.edu/marijuana/factsheets/whatiscannabis.htm#sthash.lEZ7YPbK.dpuf.

http://online.santarosa.edu/homepage/drangaves/AOLS_LecturePDFs/Cannabis_clinical_Pharmacology_Uses.pdf.

www.drugs.com.

Benzodiazepines

http://anxiety.emedtv.com/m/valium/valium-and-pregnancy.html.

http://anxiety.emedtv.com/m/valium/effects-of-valium.html.

http://www.rightdiagnosis.com/v/valium_teratogenic_agent/intro.htm.

www.rxlist.com.
www.deadiversion.usdoj.gov.

Gamma-Hydroxybutyrate (GHB)

www.drugs.com.
www.rxlist.com.
www.deadiversion.usdoj.gov.
Keltner, N., and Folks, D. Psychotropic Drugs, 4th Edition, Elsevier Mosby, 2005.

Inhalants

www.rxlist.com.
www.deadiversion.usdoj.gov.
www.drugs.com.
Keltner, N., and Folks, D. Psychotropic Drugs, 4th Edition, Elsevier Mosby, 2005.

Community Connections

http://www.aa.org. Bill W., The A.A. Service Manual combined w/12 Concepts for World Service ; 3 2014–2015 Edition. http://www.netplaces.com.

Mannion, James; 12 Steps to a Better Life. Bill W. & Company. Alcoholics Anonymous, Third Edition. 1996.

http://lighthouserecoveryinstitute.com/smart-recovery-vs-aa/.

http://www.washingtonpost.com/wp-dyn/content/article/2010/08/11/AR2010081105722.html.

www.rxlist.com.

www.deadiversion.usdoj.gov.

A.A. Website. "Historical Data: The Birth of A.A. and It's Growth in the U.S./Canada". 2015. Alcoholics Anonymous World Services, Inc. Accessed 10 Oct. 2015. http://www.aa.org/.

A.A. Website. "Twelve Steps and Twelve Traditions". 2015. Accessed 12 Oct. 2015. http://www.aa.org/pages/en_US/twelve-steps-and-twelve-traditions.

Bill W., co-founder of Alcoholics Anonymous Website. Quotations from the "Big Book." 12 April 2011. Accessed 11 Oct 2015. http://homepage.eircom.net/~recovery/big.html.

Bohlin, Erik. Website Article. "Drug Treatment Centers, Counseling, and Alcoholics Anonymous: The Pros and Cons". Accessed 13 Oct. 2015. http://www.erikbohlin.net/Treatment_Centers_AA_Counseling.htm.

Spiritual River Website. "Pros and Cons of Alcoholic Anonymous Meetings as Your Recovery Solution". 2015. Accessed 13 Oct 2015. http://www.spiritualriver.com/alcoholism/alcoholic-anonymous-meetings/.

Wilson, Bill. Alcoholics Anonymous, 1st. Edition, "How It Works", Page 58. Copyright 1939. Alcoholics Anonymous World Services, Inc.

CHAPTER SIX

OPIATE/OPIOIDS

Chapter Objectives

1. Understand the pain process and different pain mediators.
2. List various nonpharmacologic and pharmacologic medications in a pain treatment plan.
3. Recognize the opiate addiction process, symptoms, withdrawal, and treatments.

Positive Affirmations

> "What is necessary to change a person is to change his awareness of himself."
>
> —Abraham Maslow

Pharmacology

OPIATE/OPIOIDS

Opioids (Narcotics)

"Among the remedies which it has pleased Almighty God to give to man to relieve his sufferings, none is so universal and as efficacious as opium."—Sir Thomas Sydenham

Opiate is any natural sedative narcotic containing or derived from **opium.** The most common ones are **heroin, morphine, and codeine. Opioid** is any **synthetic or semisynthetic narcotic** that has opiate-like activities but is not derived from opium. Examples are **tramadol (Ultram), fentanyl, meperidine (Demerol), buprenorphine, oxymorphone, hydrocodone, oxycodone, hydromorphone (Dilaudid), and methadone.** All are reversible with naloxone and naltrexone, narcotic antagonists. For the purposes of this reading, opiates and opioids are interchangeable terms referring to the therapeutic classification of narcotics.

Pharmacologic intervention usually follows the **analgesic ladder**. Medications are given based on pain assessment, comorbid factors, and patient-specific narcotic exposure or nativity. There are three rungs on the analgesic ladder, starting with nonopioid with or without adjuvant like an antihistamine, moving next to an opioid for mild to moderate pain with or without a nonopioid and/or adjuvant, to a stronger opioid for moderate to severe pain with or without a nonopioid and/or adjuvant. Addiction is less common than many people believe in long-term chronic pain management patients. True addiction is marked by physical cravings, drug-seeking behavior, and an excessive compulsive use for euphoric effects or to avoid withdrawal symptoms. **Pseudo addiction** may develop when pain is inadequately treated. Manipulative, drug-seeking behavior stops once effective, adequate pain relief is achieved.

Opioid selections consist of **hydrocodone** (e.g., **Vicodin), oxycodone** (e.g., **OxyContin, Percocet), morphine, codeine,** and related drugs.

Hydrocodone products are the most commonly prescribed for a variety of painful conditions, including dental and injury-related pain.

Morphine is often used before and after surgical procedures to alleviate severe pain. Morphine-like opioids are well known for their addictive qualities and their ability to produce euphoria, motivating some to use opioids recreationally.

OxyContin is an oral medication used to treat moderate to severe pain through a slow, steady release of the opioid. People who abuse OxyContin may snort or inject it, increasing their risk for serious medical complications, including overdose.

Codeine in combination with **acetaminophen (APAP**) or **aspirin (ASA)** is often prescribed for mild to moderate pain. Codeine combined with the antihistamine **promethazine (Phenergan)** is a potent cough suppressant.

Diphenoxylate (Lomotil) is used for diarrhea with low addiction and abuse potential.

Selected Opioids—Synthetic Group
Meperidine (Demerol)—short acting
Methadone (Dolophine)—orally effective
Hydromorphone (Dilaudid)
Pentazocine (Talwin)
Buprenorphine (Buprenex)—partial agonist
Oxycodone (Oxycontin, Percodan, Percocet)
Hydrocodone (Vicodin, Lorcet, Norco)

In response to pain the body's natural analgesics, **endogenous endorphins** and **enkephalins** are released. They are activated by physical, chemical, emotional, or spiritual stress; pain; anticipation of pain; or threat of injury or harm. **Nociceptive neurons** are free nerve endings that are sensitive to a variety of pain stimuli. They release **Substance P** when activated. Endogenous opioids are present at brain sites. Primary pain neurotransmitters are Substance P, glutamate, GABA, norepinephrine, serotonin, and histamine. Narcotics reduce the perceptional intensity of pain signals reaching the brain. Clinical indications of opioids are analgesia, acute pulmonary edema, cough, diarrhea, and anesthesia.

They exert opiate-like effects by interacting with opiate receptors of cell membranes. Opioids act by attaching to specific proteins called **opioid receptors**, which are found in the brain, spinal cord, gastrointestinal tract, and other organs in the body. The primary classification of opioid receptors are **μ, κ, δ** (mu, kappa, and delta); however, up to 17 have been discovered, including the **ε, ι, λ,** and **ζ** (epsilon, iota, lambda, and zeta) receptors. The most important receptor is the mu receptor in the brain and spinal cord. The mu agonists mimic compounds in the body and work on multiple receptors. Opioid drugs inhibit inhibitory GABA and increase the release of dopamine. Both mechanisms are responsible for the reinforcing rewards effect.

The Pain Process

Multiple factors—physical, emotional, and spiritual—have been shown to directly stimulate nociceptors (sensory receptors that detect tissue damage and lead to the feeling of pain). As research continues, many more will likely be found. These include the following:

Globulin and protein kinases (enzymes). It has been suggested that damaged tissue releases globulin and protein kinases, which are believed to be among the most active pain-producing substances.

Arachidonic acid is one of the chemicals released during tissue damage. It is then metabolized into prostaglandin (and cytokines) by COX enzymes. The prostaglandins block the potassium efflux released from nociceptors following damage, which results in additional depolarization. This makes the nociceptors more sensitive. Aspirin and NSAIDs are effective pain-killers because it blocks the conversion of arachidonic acid to prostaglandin.

Histamine release is stimulated by **t**issue damage. The mast cells release histamine to the surrounding area. Histamine excites the nociceptors.

Nerve growth factor (NGF). Inflammation or tissue damage triggers the release of NGF. NGF then binds to TrkA receptors on the surfaces of nociceptors leading to their activation.

Substance P (SP) and calcitonin gene-related peptide (CGRP) are released by injury. Inflammation of tissue damage also results in SP and CGRP release, which excites nociceptors. Both peptides produce vasodilation, which results in the spread of edema around the initial damage.

Potassium-K+. Most tissue damage results in an increase in extracellular K+. There is a good correlation between pain intensity and local K+ concentration.

Serotonin (5-HT), acetylcholine (ACh), low pH (acidic) solution, and ATP. These substances are released with tissue damage.

Muscle spasm and lactic acid. Not only can some headaches result from muscle spasms of smooth muscle but stretching of a ligament can also elicit pain. When muscles are hyperactive or when blood flow to a muscle is blocked, lactic acid concentration increases, and pain is induced. The greater the rate of tissue metabolism, the more rapidly the pain appears.

Pharmacologic Medications in Pain Management

- NSAIDS (ibuprofen, naproxen), acetaminophen, aspirin
- Antidepressants (amitriptyline, fluoxetine, duloxetine)
- Antiseizure meds, neuromodulators (gabapentin, valproic acid, pregabalin, pramipexole)
- Muscle relaxants (cyclobenzaprine, clonazepam)

- Local salves (lidocaine, capsaicin)
- Analgesic ladder—weak to stronger opioids (tramadol)

Nonpharmacologic Pain Management Techniques

- Distraction—Ice, heat, TV, read, visiting
- Relaxation—Breathing, yoga, tapes, music
- Massage, physical therapy, exercise, strength training
- Cognitive behavioral therapy, biofeedback
- Acupuncture, acupressure, healthy diet
- Imagery, aromatherapy

The side effect profile of opioids includes sedation, rash, itching, hives (especially with morphine and codeine), gastrointestinal upset, nausea, vomiting, constipation, a sense of euphoria, dizziness, and headache. Dose-depending adverse effects produce mental confusion, difficulty breathing or swallowing, respiratory depression, seizures, and irregular heartbeat (arrhythmia).

Opioid drugs demonstrate tolerance and cross-tolerance with other drugs in the same class.

Some people experience a euphoric response to opioid medications since these drugs also affect the brain regions involved in reward. Those who abuse opioids seek to intensify the euphoric experience. Even a single large dose can cause severe respiratory depression and death. Opioids must not be used with other substances that depress the central nervous system, such as alcohol, antihistamines, barbiturates, benzodiazepines, or general anesthetics. This combination increases the risk of life-threatening respiratory depression.

Common Opioid Side Effects

- Constipation
- Mental clouding, fatigue
- Nausea, vomiting
- Itching, sweating
- Urinary retention

Acute opioid overdose intoxication causes low blood pressure and respiration depression, fixed pinpoint pupils, depressed sensorium, coma, and pulmonary edema. Rapid reversal occurs after administration of a **pure opioid antagonist**: **Naloxone (Narcan), Naltrexone**, or a **mixed agonist-antagonist, Nalorphine.**

Properly managed, short-term medical use of opioid analgesics rarely causes addiction—characterized by compulsive drug seeking and use despite serious adverse consequences. Using nonsteroidal anti-inflammatory drugs (NSAIDs) in combination with opioids can reduce the opioid dose needed by up to 40%. There is a maximum dose for each NSAID and acetaminophen. However, narcotics do not have a ceiling dose. Regular (e.g., several times a day, for several weeks or more) or longer term use or abuse of opioids can lead to physical dependence and, in some cases, addiction. The individual molecular structure of opioids is responsible for the different duration of action, onset of action, metabolic breakdown, and opioid metabolism and elimination. Opioid dependence can develop with ongoing administration, leading to a withdrawal syndrome with abrupt discontinuation.

Reinforcing pharmacologic properties of narcotics include pain relief, change or elevation of mood, relief of tension, fear, anxiety, and the production of feelings of peace, euphoria, and tranquility via increase DA activity. Symptoms of use or abuse are drowsiness, droopy eyelids, pinpoint pupils, lethargy, needle marks, loss of appetite, and signs of withdrawal.

Abstinence or withdrawal symptoms of opioids are related to the half-life of the specific agent. Symptoms usually develop within two to 48 hours and peak at about 72 hours. They include chills, hot flashes, restless sleep, piloerection on the skin (cold turkey), rhinorrhea, drowsiness, lacrimation, mydriasis, sneezing, yawning, cramping, vomiting, diarrhea, anorexia, increased blood pressure, pulse, temperature, and drug craving. If left untreated, physical withdrawal may continue up to 7–10 days; psychological dependence continues for longer of forever. Cardiovascular collapse may be the consequence if withdrawal is severe without supportive treatment.

Detoxification is the first step in drug abuse treatment. Opioid abuse treatment programs include the substitution of one opioid, such as methadone or buprenorphine, for the abused drug. These substitutes, when given orally, produce no euphoria and eliminate craving for heroin and reduce exposure to risk to HIV and hepatitis. The long-acting opioids stabilize the physiological effects and encourage contact with support staff. Methadone has a mild withdrawal. There are few damaging effects on organs with prolonged use. Compared with methadone, buprenorphine is longer acting, has a milder withdrawal and neonatal withdrawal, and can be prescribed in a physician's office. When combined with naloxone, abuse potential is reduced. Opioid antagonists are effective in blocking the opioid receptors so that self-administered narcotics have no effect. The most successful treatment approaches are multidimensional ones.

Opium

The word "opium" comes from the Greek opos (juice) and opion (poppy juice). Opium is recognized for its narcotic and medicinal properties used to regulate constipation, sleep, and panacea. The principle active ingredient, **morphenine**, deadens pain, produces ecstasy, induces sleep, and reduces distress. It can be smoked, swallowed, sniffed, rubbed, or injected. Opium is highly addictive with a high potential for abuse. Prior to this knowledge, opium was found in multiple over-the -counter medicines—products that were used to quiet crying babies, calm frayed nerves, and restore health to millions. Today, opium is a narcotic or opiate, which is a therapeutic classification of pain-reducing drugs that produces a relaxed dreamlike state; moderately high doses often induce sleep. Opiates create a clouding of consciousness. Regular use of any of the narcotics can lead to a withdrawal syndrome different than that of depressants and characterized by diarrhea, cramps, chills, and profuse sweating.

Heroin

Heroin is an opioid drug and has been classified as a Schedule I drug, highly addictive with a high potential for abuse. Heroin is derived from morphine, which can be extracted from the opium poppy plant. It can be up to 2–3 times more potent than the morphine. This addictive drug can be snorted, smoked, or, most commonly, injected. Pure heroin is white but is often mixed with other substances. Heroin is sold on the streets today under many different names such as smack, H, junk, and horse. Street heroin is found in a powder form that is usually white to brownish in color. Black tar heroin is another form that gets its name from looking like roofing tar or coal.

Most heroin users call it "the rush." It is the high or euphoric feeling that the person gets after administration of the drug. Heroin is converted back into morphine that binds to opioid receptors. Opioid receptors are found in many areas of the brain and in the body; many are involved with the person's perception of pain. Injection of the drug is most common because it gives the person that rush much quicker than smoking or snorting it.

The effects of heroin are the same with any of the administrations: rapid onset and a duration lasting only a few hours. It has been reported that once the person has injected heroin and felt the euphoric rush, he or she experiences dry mouth with warm flushed skin, heavy extremities, and clouded mental functions that can result in an alternately wakeful and drowsy state. Additional effects include respiratory depression, constricted pupils, and nausea. Heroin overdoses are often due to suppression of breathing, which affects the amount of oxygen that goes to your brain. If a person does have an overdose, he or she is in high risk of muscle spasms, hypotension, convulsions, slow/ shallow breathing, coma, and, possibly, death.

The most common long-term result of using heroin is tolerance; the user must use more of the drug to achieve the same intensity. Other long-term results are dependence and addiction. Some studies have shown deterioration of parts of the brain from heroin use. This affects the decision-making process, self-regulation of behavior, and responses to situations. Drug dependence continues in order to avoid withdrawal symptoms such as drug cravings, restlessness, muscle and bone pain, diarrhea and vomiting, cold flashes, kicking movements, and many other symptoms. Some of these symptoms can start as soon as a couple of hours after initial administration, and major withdrawal symptoms can peak between 48–72 hours.

With injectable heroin, users have concurrent serious health issues that can develop by sharing contaminated needs, including HIV/AIDS, hepatitis, and toxic reactions to the drug's impurities. The impurities in heroin when injected can clog blood vessels that lead to the lungs, liver, kidneys, or brain. Clogging these blood vessels can cause serious or permanent damage to many vital organs. Collapsed veins, inflammation of the heart lining and valves, spontaneous abortion, abscesses, and pneumonia are other complications that users can develop. Pneumonia often becomes a complication due to the poor health of the user and the effects heroin has on breathing. Heroin use while pregnant can lead to low birth weight, which is a very important risk factor for delays in development. There is a possibility that the infant will be born physically dependent on heroin and could suffer from a drug withdrawal syndrome that would require hospitalization if the mother is using the drug often.

There are many different heroin treatments that include **harm reduction therapy**, behavioral therapy, and medications.

Synthetic Opiates

Methadone, also known as **Dolophine**, among other brand names, is a synthetic opioid. It is used medically as a pain medication managing severe chronic pain due to its long duration of action and strong analgesic effect. Methadone maintenance therapy is indicated in the treatment for heroin and other opioid dependency. The withdrawal from opioids and opiates is a physically painful experience. Methadone's chemical structure is an analog of morphine and heroin; therefore, it acts on the same opioid receptors. Methadone does not cause the same initial euphoric rush as heroin and other drugs. There are, however, many adverse side effects from methadone, including sedation, diarrhea, nausea, and vomiting.

Studies have shown that **methadone maintenance therapy (MMT)** reduces or eliminates the cravings for opiates, reduces the death rates and criminality associated with heroin use, and promotes physical and emotional health. The treatment of opiate-dependent persons with methadone maintenance therapy is prescribed to individuals who wish to abstain from illicit drug use but have failed to maintain abstinence from opiates for significant periods. The duration of methadone maintenance can be for months or even years. **Methadone reduction programs** are suitable for addicted persons who wish to stop using drugs altogether. The length of the reduction program will depend on the starting dose and speed of reduction; this varies from clinic to clinic and from person to person. In addition, enrollment in a methadone program has the potential to reduce the transmission of infectious diseases associated with opiate injection, such as hepatitis and HIV.

When used appropriately, methadone maintenance has been found to be medically safe and nonsedating. It is also indicated for pregnant women addicted to opiates; however, only if the benefit clearly outweighs the risk to the fetus. Prolonged use of methadone can result in physical dependency in the neonate. Methadone maintenance therapy, under doctor's supervision, is a safe alternative to using illicit drugs such as heroin or other opiate-based street drugs while pregnant. Methadone maintenance eliminates cravings for opiates and blocks the effects of opioids as well as prevents the onset of withdrawal. It reduces the stress on the fetus from repeated withdrawal and the seemingly never-ending cycle of opioid intoxication and withdrawal, which can trigger spontaneous abortion or premature labor.

Babies born to mothers on methadone will present with withdrawal symptoms, including fussiness, restlessness, lack of appetite and sleep, fever, vomiting, diarrhea, trembling, high pitch crying, and be difficult to console. Symptoms may not present for 72 hours or up until one week after birth. These babies are at a greater risk for **sudden infant death syndrome (SIDS)**. They recover best with low stimuli environments and need to be kept swaddled, cradled, and rocked for comfort.

Methadone and buprenorphine work by binding to the same cell receptors as heroin. **Buprenorphin**e, combined with **naloxone and naltrexone**, help block the opioid receptors that prevent the drug from having an effect. For a gradual withdrawal, oral administration is recommended for these drugs. Methadone is highly regulated in the US and has been used in treatment for over a quarter of a century. There are certified treatment programs that are approved to use oral methadone to aid in the detox and maintenance of a user. Most users have daily treatment and follow-ups in these programs.

Buprenorphine/naloxone (Suboxone) is an opioid agonist used in pain management and opiate dependence. Treatments can be more acceptable to patients and can be done in an authorized physician's office, making it a great outpatient maintenance therapy. This drug reduces craving and increases success in abstinence programs.

Naltrexone has a long-acting injection that is used for following up opiate detox. Naltrexone is a pure opioid antagonist, which will only be administered to patients who have been opioid free for seven to ten days due to possible withdrawal symptoms if the body is not opioid free. With these combined therapies, patients have the potential to become functioning members of society

LAAM (levo-alpha-acetylmethadol), or **levomethadyl acetate (Orlaam),** is a longer acting alternative to methadone to reduce opioid cravings. It is given three times a week and is preferred by some patients to the daily methadone dosing. Treatment has been shown to be comparable to methadone treatment regarding decreased opioid use; however, retention rates are higher for patients treated with methadone. The longer the treatment duration with LAAN, the better the associated outcomes. Monitoring cardiovascular function with an ECG is required.

Alpha Omega

"My name is Estella, and I was born addicted to heroin. This unfortunate experience happened because my mother was a heroin addict. I am 20 years old now, and I want to share my story with the hope that it will help other addicts like my mom. When I was about 16 years old, my mom told me that I was born addicted to heroin. At first I was shocked, but I am very proud of her that she was so brave to share the truth with me. She has been clean now for 20 years, and is trying to help others who are still suffering from addiction.

"When I was conceived, my mother had just dropped out of high school and had run away from home. She was 16 years old and didn't have anywhere to live except on the streets. After living one week on the streets, she learned that the only way to survive was to sell her body for money and for acceptance. She soon became pregnant with me and didn't know it until she was three months pregnant. My mother was a beautiful Latina young woman. She had long straight black hair and large soft brown eyes. I don't think she knew how beautiful she was, but she soon became very popular with the men in the neighborhood. Everyone called her by her nickname, "Chi-Chi." She didn't like her real name because it reminded her of her father who used to sexually abuse her. As she got older, she would fight him, but he was much bigger and stronger, so he would only hurt her more. That is the reason why she finally ran away from home. I think maybe she thought that the streets would be better than taking any more abuse from him. I don't think she had any idea how difficult being homeless was going to be for her.

"Right after I was conceived, my mother started using heroin. Heroin eased my mother's emotional pain that she had been in most of her childhood and helped her to handle the stress of being on the streets and sleeping with strange men. I became addicted because the heroin she ingested traveled to my growing embryo through the placenta. My mom snorted it, and it's probably good that she did, or I may not have had a chance to live. I guess I was "lucky" in this area, but my mother didn't eat very well, so I was very underweight when I was born. My mother's water broke early, and I was born a month early, weighing only 3.5 pounds and measuring seven inches long. Luckily a nice man helped my mom get to the hospital when her water broke, and they rushed us to the emergency room. They had to do a cesarean section to safely remove my little body, and I was rushed to the baby intensive care unit. I could not breathe on my own for a while because my lungs were not fully developed yet. It was really a miracle that I survived at all.

"When I was born, I had what is called **neonatal abstinence syndrome (NAS).** This basically means that I was presenting with symptoms of sudden withdrawal of a maternally transferred opioid. I had all of the symptoms, including poor feeding, uncoordinated and constant sucking, vomiting, diarrhea, dehydration, poor weight gain, sweating, fever, temperature instability, and nasal stuffiness. I also presented with neurologic excitability, such as tremors, irritability, increased wakefulness, high-pitched crying, frequent yawning, and sneezing. I had to be treated with methadone for several weeks and so did my mother. After almost a month of intensive care in the hospital, we were released to a long-term residential drug treatment program. This was where my mom was finally able to get the love and support she needed to stay clean. I had many learning and behavioral disabilities, but the staff at Rosa House helped me to get into the kinds of programs that would help me to learn. I feel like I was one of the lucky few because many babies and their mothers die in childbirth if the mother was a chronic user like mine. I guess I was meant to share my story. I hope it helps you or someone you love somehow."—Anonymous

Critical Thinking

"Our stories disclose in a general way what we used to be like, what happened, and what we are like now. If you have decided you want what we have and are willing to go to any length to get it—then you are ready to take certain steps. At some of these we balked. We thought we could find an easier, softer way. But we could not. Half-measures availed us nothing. Here are the steps we took, which are suggested as a program of recovery (The Big Book, 3rd Edition, William G. Wilson, pages 58 to 59.) I can't tell you how many times I have heard this very reading and how many people whose lives have been changed dramatically due to this simple statement. The number of alcoholics finding solutions to their dilemma are growing rapidly due to the fact that the 12 Steps, in fact, do work. The abuse behavior or substance of choice does not matter. There are over 130 different 12-Step Programs that help all types of addiction.

"I was 18 the first time I tried to get sober. I had been struggling with binge drinking for some time and ended up getting a DUI. After that, I was introduced to treatment as well as the 12-Step Programs. Alcoholism was never discussed in my family. It was the little secret that no one cared to deal with or discuss. It wasn't until I went to treatment that I realized I wasn't alone and that there were, in fact, many people just like me; normal, loving, caring, funny, and smart people who also struggled with addiction. This is one of the things that makes AA so successful; you have all this shame and darkness that you don't want anyone to see, and then you attend an AA meeting and realize, 'Wow, I am not alone. It's not only me.' 'Yeah, me too' is one of the most powerful statements that people can say to one another to be able to connect on a deeper level.

"I have heard it said many times in the rooms (I am paraphrasing) that alcoholics are like soldiers who have gone to battle together, and we have a comradery that no one, other than the other alcoholic, can understand; we have gone through hell and made it to the other side. There are as many treatment modalities as there are different types of people. It doesn't necessarily have to be one type of thing that works for one person. There are many different avenues to recovery as well as to finding a solution that works for you. However, there generally has to be a shift for most people, a so-called 'hitting bottom,' that pushes people to desire a change to better their lives. I think the desire to change is a beautiful thing to watch in people: to grow, to change, to adapt, to overcome. There is nothing more inspiring to me than when a person finds that what he or she is doing isn't working anymore and actually takes the action to change that. The human spirit is awe inspiring when it comes to resiliency."—Anonymous

Methadone Maintenance

"Having struggled with a heroin addiction for many years, I wholeheartedly believe in harm reduction therapy. I had tried many times to kick my heroin habit and was unable to do so. I was introduced to a methadone maintenance clinic in my late twenties, early thirties, and was grateful for the support and education I received at this clinic with regard to the disease of addiction. Before getting on methadone, I had been arrested, was completely unemployable, and was having a hard time taking care of my basic needs. The structure that was offered at this clinic as well as the accountability helped me turn my life around.

"I met many women, some of whom were pregnant, who were going through the same life experiences as me, and they were able to turn their lives around. They even received additional help through the very agencies they feared would take their babies. They were able to get the prenatal care that they would otherwise not have been able to receive. They found support in each other at the meetings they were required to attend, and they, too, were able to stay clean, get jobs, and support their families. They were able to begin to show up in their own lives both financially and emotionally due to this harm reduction therapy and that helped save their lives as well as the lives of their unborn babies.

"So, although research shows that babies born chemically dependent to methadone suffer for a short time with withdrawal, I believe without the support offered through these treatment programs, a short-term physical problem for the mother and fetus could turn into a lifelong struggle for all. Also, methadone should be used as a temporary solution, and parents have a responsibility to work towards a clean, sober, and safe environment for their children."—Anonymous

OPIATE/OPIOIDS

Analgesic Pharmacology:

https://www.youtube.com/watch?v=LLv29S7Hm3U

How Opioids Work:

https://www.youtube.com/watch?v=BKMlHNqlQsM

Pharmacology of Opioids/Opioid Receptors:

https://www.youtube.com/watch?v=YCz5A8ZkavM

Pain and Opioids 3D Animation:

https://www.youtube.com/watch?v=paAzzwZi3vk

Opioid Tolerance:

https://www.youtube.com/watch?v=W2QjbdYfakg

OPIUM

Where Does Opium Come From:

https://www.youtube.com/watch?v=2AFUPv7DRxs

HEROIN

Heroin and Methadone Effects on the Brain:

https://www.youtube.com/watch?v=qpzPZRm2S98

Heroin:

http://www.drugfreeworld.org/real-life-stories/heroin.html

Reversing a Heroin Overdose:

https://www.youtube.com/watch?v=UASuPWTobvI

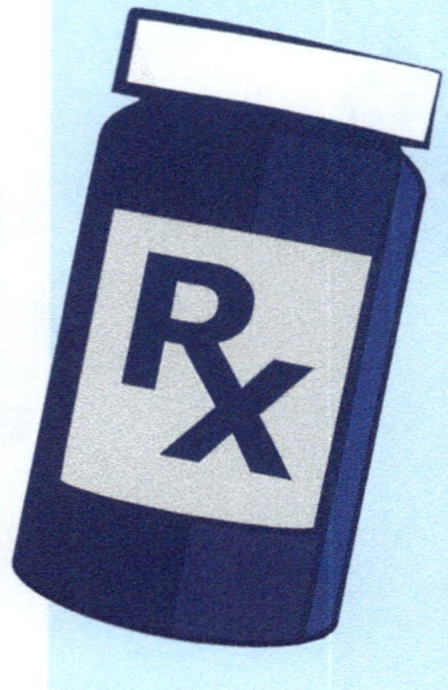

Drug Sandbox

Important Words to Know!

Opiate
Opium
Heroin
Morphine
Codeine
Opioid
Synthetic or Semisynthetic Narcotic
Tramadol (Ultram®)
Fentanyl,
Meperidine (Demerol®)
Buprenorphine
Oxymorphone
Hydrocodone
Oxycodone
Hydromorphone (Dilaudid®)
Methadone
Analgesic Ladder
Pseudo Addiction
Hydrocodone
Oxycodone
Morphine
Codeine
Acetaminophen (APAP)
Aspirin (ASA)
Promethazine (Phenergan®)
Diphenoxylate (Lomotil®)
Endogenous Endorphins
Enkephalins
Nociceptive Neurons
Substance P
Opioid Receptors
Acute Opioid Overdose Intoxication
Pure Opioid Antagonist
Naloxone (Narcan®)
Naltrexone
Mixed Agonist-Antagonist, Nalorphine.
Reinforcing Pharmacologic Properties
Abstinence or Withdrawal
Morphenine
Harm Reduction Therapy
Methadone
Dolophine
Methadone Maintenance Therapy (MMT)
Methadone Reduction Programs
Sudden Infant Death Syndrome (SIDS)
Buprenorphine
Levomethadyl Acetate (ORLAAM)

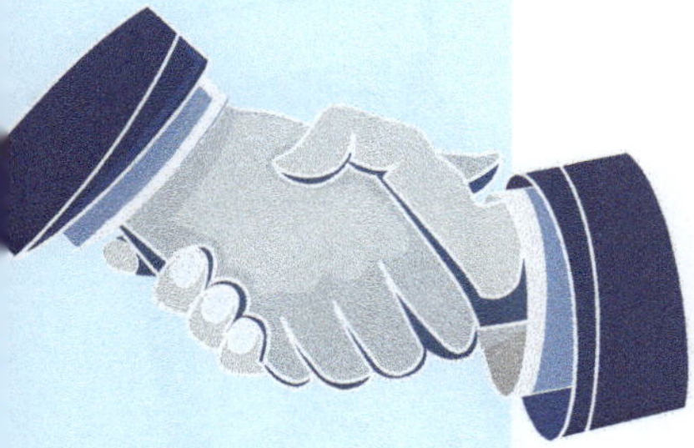

Community Connections

NARCOTICS ANONYMOUS: MORE GOOD THAN BAD

"Narcotics Anonymous saved my life. I was introduced to Narcotics Anonymous through a treatment facility I entered for a heroin addiction I had been struggling with for 15 years

"Narcotics Anonymous (NA) is a drug addiction recovery support group based on the 12 Steps of Alcoholics Anonymous (AA). NA groups are made up of people who meet regularly to help each other stop using drugs and stay drug free. NA has replaced the word 'alcohol' with 'addiction' in AA's 12 Steps to reflect the disease concept of addiction. Through this 12-Step Program, NA provides a recovery process and support group for people who have a desire to put an end to their substance abuse. Although NA has existed since the late 1940s, there is a lack of scientific evidence that the program is any more effective than doing nothing; however, my first-hand participation and observations of the NA program indicate its effectiveness.

"NA provides many benefits for its members, but there are a number of flaws in the structure of the program. And even though NA may not be perfect, there is no disputing that NA has saved many addicts' lives. The most obvious flaw in NA is its all-inclusion policy. Anybody can attend meetings and participate in the program. Although at first glance, this may appear to be a good policy, it creates an environment where predators can target vulnerable individuals. Many people receive 'a nudge from the judge' to attend NA meetings. Criminals are often required to attend NA meetings as part of their sentences. It is not uncommon to have 5–10 criminals attending any given meeting, but they have no desire to discontinue using drugs or changing their behavior. NA members make the assumption that a person has good intentions if he or she is attending meetings. I know of people who suffered deeply as a result of making this assumption.

"Another area of concern with NA, and most 12-Step Programs, for that matter, is the incestuous sexual behavior among members. It is quite common for addicts to date each other. This isn't necessarily harmful for addicts who have reached a stable state in their recovery. The problem arises when a member with time and experience in the program preys on a newer member. This type of behavior is called '13th Stepping.' Addicts normally arrive in NA with little or no self-respect and a poorly developed sense of personal boundaries.

A newcomer usually suffers from low self-esteem, which causes him or her to believe that any attention is good attention. This dynamic makes a newcomer easy pickings for the manipulative old timer. When things go south in this type of relationship, the newcomer often relapses because he or she hasn't yet built a foundation of recovery to fall back on.

"One cannot discuss the drawbacks of NA without addressing the assertion that recovery is dependent on a member having faith in God or a Higher Power. The program's fundamental adherence in the belief of a Higher Power is a difficult pill to swallow, especially for humanists or atheists. While this higher power is sometimes interpreted as the program itself, this reliance on an outside power to guide the process may not be a comfortable notion for everyone. I struggle quite a bit with the Higher Power concept and am turned off by God-centric talk in meetings. It doesn't matter what members call 'it,' we just need to know that we are not the center of the universe. I found relief in realizing that I could turn over control to something other than myself. That something is a group of people whom I trust, and I consider a group consciousness to be my Higher Power. What a gift!

"There are no trained counselors, therapists, or social workers providing treatment in NA. Any addict who has worked the 12 Steps can be a sponsor. A sponsor is essentially any member willing to guide a newer member through the process of recovery. The quality of a sponsor is often determined by the luck of the draw. It is suggested that members choose a sponsor who exhibits qualities that they themselves would like to develop. Common complaints about a sponsor range from hypocrisy, control issues, and, sometimes, abusive behavior. A sponsor is, in fact, just another sick addict.

"One of the best things about Narcotics Anonymous is that anyone, and I mean anyone, can join. NA is the place where any outcast can become part of a group. Addicts often use drugs to fill the void of not having human connections. In NA, nobody is excluded from participating. The only requirement for membership is the desire to stay clean. There simply isn't an objective method for measuring a person's desire to stop using, so everyone is welcome. Many people come to Narcotics Anonymous with absolutely no pro-social skills because they have lived in isolation for many years. NA might be the only public group where such individuals are freely accepted for who they are. I arrived in Narcotics Anonymous with a desire to stay out of prison. I didn't imagine that I would become a socially acceptable, responsible member of society as result of participating in the program.

"An honest, recovering addict will admit that his or her first few years of recovery are spent in an aroused sexual state. Perhaps there is a pharmacological basis for this phenomenon, or maybe addicts seek sex because it is another method of getting high. Either way, it is much better for two recovering addicts to hook up than it is for a recovering addict to get together with a person who uses. I know many happy, healthy couples that met in NA. The better NA fellowships encourage the men to stick with men and the women to stick with women, especially in early recovery. Members often report finding their first spiritually healthy partner in 12-Step Programs.

"I wouldn't suggest taking legal or medical advice from a random member of Narcotics Anonymous. NA does not employ any type of professionals. There is, however, value in one addict helping another to stay clean. Only an addict can truly relate to another addict's experience. This is the reason that sponsorship is so effective: a newer member can draw from the wealth of wisdom that a seasoned member of NA possesses, and we usually feel comfortable sharing our histories with people who have done the types of things we have done. I did therapy for almost a decade and had marginal success. I processed deep-seated trauma with my sponsor in less than six months. It was easier to talk to him because he had experienced the same kind of trauma that I had.

"NA is not perfect, and it can be argued that it is a cult. I would still recommend it to anyone who believes he or she may have an addiction to drugs. I have witnessed transformations that can be described as nothing less than a miracle. NA has turned me into a person that I can respect. I do, however, caution newer members to keep their guard up and to trust their instincts with people they meet in meetings. Most of us were villains before we got in recovery; some of us recovered and became spiritual, moral, and ethical as a result of working the Steps. Narcotics Anonymous saves lives, but it is not for everyone."—Anonymous

End Of Chapter Review Questions

Multiple Choices: Select the best answer from the choices given:

1. The use of opioids for noncancer pain:
    a. Is a reasonable option for some patients
    b. Is never appropriate
    c. Is illegal
    d. Always leads to addiction

2. Opioids should not be combined with:
    a. NSAIDs
    b. Antibiotics
    c. Barbiturates
    d. Acetaminophen
    e. Biofeedback

3. Addiction is associated with:
    a. Physical craving
    b. Excessive use
    c. Compulsive use
    d. All of the above

4. Common side effects of opioids include all of the following except:
    a. Diarrhea
    b. Mental clouding, fatigue
    c. Nausea, vomiting
    d. Itching, sweating
    e. Urinary retention

5. Nonpharmacologic pain management techniques include all of the following except:
    a. Distraction—Ice, heat, TV, read, visiting
    b. Relaxation—Breathing, yoga, tapes, music
    c. Massage, physical therapy, exercise, strength training
    d. Cognitive behavioral therapy, biofeedback
    e. Acetaminophen

6. Pharmacologic medications in pain management are:
    a. NSAIDS (ibuprofen, naproxen), acetaminophen, aspirin
    b. Antidepressants (amitriptyline, fluoxetine, duloxetine)
    c. Antiseizure meds, neuromodulators (gabapentin, valproic acid, pregabalin, pramipexole)
    d. Muscle relaxants (cyclobenzaprine, clonazepam)
    e. Local salves (lidocaine, capsaicin)
    f. All of the above

7. An NA recovery client falls and sprains an anklSelect the best medication treatment recommendation:
    a. Meperidine
    b. Methadone
    c. Motrin
    d. Vicodin
    e. Norco

8. Which of the following statements is false regarding OxyContin?
    a. It is an oral medication used to treat moderate to severe pain.
    b. It is a slow, steady release of the opioid.
    c. People who abuse OxyContin may snort or inject it.
    d. An overdose is reversed with flumazenil.

9. In response to pain, the body's natural analgesics are:
    a. Endorphins and enkephalins.
    b. Endogenous hydrocodone
    c. Histamine
    d. Arachidonic acid
    e. Protein kinase

10. Rapid reversal of acute opioid overdose intoxication involves administration of:
    a. Analog of morphine and heroin
    b. Naloxone
    c. Naltrexone
    d. B and C
    e. None of the above—only supportive care

11. Symptoms of an opioid overdose include all of the following except:
    a. Low blood pressure
    b. Respiratory excitation
    c. Fixed pinpoint pupils
    d. Depressed sensorium
    e. Pulmonary edema

12. Which of the following is false regarding abstinence or withdrawal symptoms of opioids?
    a. Are related to the half-life of the specific agent
    b. Usually develops within the 2 to 48 hours and peaks at about 72 hours
    c. Symptom of piloerection on the skin
    d. Anticholinergic symptoms of dry eyes, nose, and mouth
    e. Are caused by anorexia

13. Studies have shown that methadone maintenance therapy (MMT):
    a. Reduces or eliminates the cravings for opiates
    b. Increases the death rates
    c. Increases criminality
    d. Detracts from physical and emotional health

14. Buprenorphine/naloxone (Suboxone):
    a. Is an opioid agonist used in pain management and opiate dependence
    b. Is a benzodiazepine agonist used in pain management and opiate dependence
    c. Is a benzodiazepine antagonist used in pain management and opiate dependence
    d. Is an aversion therapy drug that increases cravings

15. An opiate is any natural sedative narcotic containing or derived from:
    a. OxyContin
    b. Oxycodone
    c. Substance P
    d. Opium
    e. Serotonin

16. An opioid is any synthetic or semisynthetic narcotic that has opiate-like activities and is not derived from:
    a. OxyContin
    b. Oxycodone
    c. Substance P
    d. Opium
    e. Serotonin

17. The first step in drug abuse treatment is:
    a. Methadone maintenance therapy
    b. Detoxification
    c. Aversion therapy
    d. Harm reduction therapy
    e. Heroin

18. Heroin use is associated with:
    a. Tolerance
    b. Dependence
    c. Addiction
    d. Deterioration of parts of the brain
    e. All of the above

19. Heroin is derived from:
    a. Methadone
    b. Methylamphetamine
    c. Morphine
    d. Meperidine
    e. None of the above

20. In the pain process, multiple factors have been show to lead to the feeling of pain. They are:
    a. Physical
    b. Emotional
    c. Spiritual
    d. Only A
    e. Only B
    f. All of the above

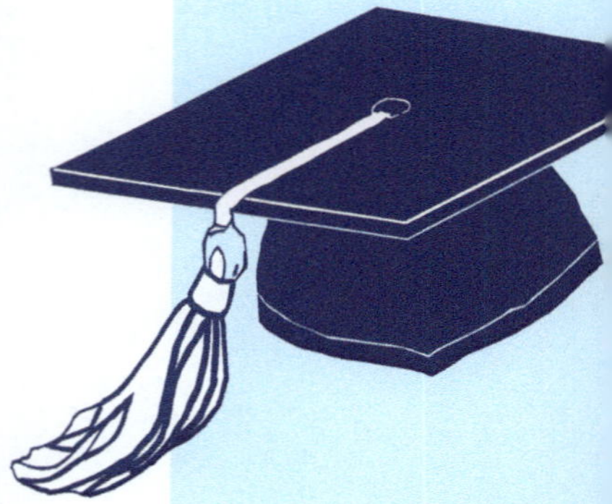

Applications: Assessment of Usage and Relevance

1. Conner is a 56-year-old male client who has had chronic pain from degenerative disc disease for six years. He has tried all the over-the-counter drugs at maximum recommended dosages and is no longer getting relief from them.
   a. What are the analgesic drug classes and MOA of each available to him?
   b. What are the indications and contraindications of each analgesic class?
   c. What is the analgesic ladder? Recommend a treatment plan using the analgesic ladder.
   d. Educate on the top two side effects of each drug you recommend. What medications do you recommend for him and why?

2. Roberta is a 32-year-old female client with back pain caused by osteoarthritis of the spine. She has been taking acetaminophen without relief. She has started on hydrocodone/APAP and pentazocine.
   a. What are the possible side effects?
   b. What are some patient education guidelines for taking the medication?
   c. Which nonpharmaceutical treatments should she receive?
   d. What is abstinence syndrome? How does is occur?

3. Daniel is a 51-year-old male client who is post-op bowel resection to relieve an obstruction. He complains of pain around his incision. He has been in recovery for five years and attends regular AA and NA meetings as a sponsor. His chart meds are Percocet, Meperidine, and Tylenol.
   a. Percocet: What are the mechanism of action, duration of action, efficacy, and three potential side effects?
   b. Meperidine: What are the mechanism of action, duration of action, efficacy, potential side effects, and drug interactions of concern?
   c. Tylenol: What are the mechanism of action, duration of action, efficacy, potential side effects, and drug interactions of concern?
   d. The client will be discharged with Vicodin 5/500 two tablets four times a day #240. Why is maintenance Vicodin a potential problem at this dose?
   e. Discuss options for pain management.
   f. List some patient education issues to address.

4. Outline the history of opium use from ancient times through the Opium Wars and in the American Civil War's aftermath.

5. Explain the history of legal actions as they affected the use of opioids and the use of opium.

6. Describe the mechanism as how opiates effect or control the pain sensorium in the body.

7. What are the potential side effects, short term and long term, of opiate use?

8. What are the signs of acetaminophen and aspirin overdose? What patient education would you give a client regarding the risks?

KEY

1. A	6. F	11. B	16. D
2. C	7. C	12. D	17. B
3. D	8. D	13. A	18. E
4. A	9. A	14. A	19. C
5. E	10. D	15. D	20. F

REFERENCES

Heroin

Fletcher, Bennett F., ed. The Implementation of Innovative Approaches. {New York}: Praeger, 1994. Print.

Anderson, Leigh. *Heroin: Effects, Addiction & Treatment Options.* 2014. http://www.drugs.com/illicit/heroin.html.

Johnson, Andrew, ed. "MMT for Clients Who Are Pregnant." Center for Addiction and Mental Health. CAMH, 27 Apr. 2009. Web. 14 Sept. 2015. https://www.camh.ca/.

"Medication Assisted Treatment Tip # 43." SAMHSA. HHS, 1 Jan. 2005. Web. 14 Sept. 2015. https://.www.ncbi.nlm.nih.gov/books]https://.www.ncbi.nlm.nih.gov/books.

What are the treatments for heroin addiction? | National Institute on Drug Abuse (NIDA). www.drugabuse.gov.
Methadone Detox | Withdrawal Pain | Methadone Treatment www.novusdetox.com.
Methadone Addiction and Side Effects | Pat Moore Foundation www.patmoorefoundation.com.
www.rxlist.com.
www.deadiversion.usdoj.gov.

Portrayal Paradigm

"Religious Roots: Bill Wilson Writes the Twelve Steps." Web. 15 Sept. 2015.
"12-Step Success Rates." Web. 15 Sept. 2015.
Smith, Robert Holbrook, and Bill W. The Big Book of Alcoholics Anonymous: The Story of How Many Thousands of Men and Women Have Recovered from Alcoholism. United States: Lark, 2013. Print.

Community Connections

Narcotics Anonymous. "What is the Narcotics Anonymous Program?" (PDF). Narcotics Anonymous. NA White Booklet (PDF). Narcotics Anonymous World Services, Inc. Archived from the original (PDF) on February 6, 2007, reproduced in Who, What, How, and Why. Narcotics Anonymous World Services, Inc.

CHAPTER SEVEN

HALLUCINOGENS

Chapter Objectives

1. Compose a reflection on the concepts empathogen and entactogen.
2. Appraise the differences between the neurotransmitter categories of hallucinogens and provide an example of each.
3. Discuss the process involved in hallucinogen intoxication and addiction treatment.

Positive Affirmations

> "Whatever you do, if you do it sincerely, will eventually become a bridge to your wholeness, a good ship that carries you through the darkness."
>
> —Carl Jung

Pharmacology

HALLUCINOGENS

Hallucinogens, referred to as **psychomimetics or psychedelics**, alter perception, enhance awareness, and can cause terrifying psychotic-like reactions. Natural hallucinogenic substances include **mescaline/peyote** from cactus and

psilocybin from mushrooms. Manufactured, synthetic, or semisynthetic substances include **lysergic acid diethylamide (LSD)**, **phencyclidine (PCP)**, **dimethyltryptamine (DMT)**, **methylenedioxyamphetamine (MDA)**, and **2.5-dimethoxy-4-methylamphetamine (STP)**.

Psychedelics and hallucinogens comprise several types categorized by the neurotransmitter they affect: **acetylcholine** psychedelics, **catecholamine**-like, **serotonin**-like, and **glutaminergic NMDA.** Psychoactive drugs in this group are also termed empathogen and entactogen, named for the paradigm experience of oneness, emotional openness, and communion produced upon use. LSD, DMT, and psilocybin are serotonin-like hallucinogens. Mescaline, MDA, and Ecstasy are norepinephrine-like hallucinogens.

Scopolamine and **hyoscyamine** are examples of anticholinergic psychedelics. They block acetylcholine (Ach) receptors in the peripheral nervous system, producing **anticholinergic syndrome**. "Hot as a hare, blind as a bat, dry as a bone, red as a beet, mad as a hen" is a metaphor to recall the effects. Plant sources of ACh psychedelics include Solanaceae, family of potato and tomatoes; Atropa belladonna, deadly nightshade; Datura stramonium, jimsonweed; and Mandragora officinarum, mandrake.

Mescaline, **Ecstasy (MDMA)**, **DOM**, **MMDA**, **myristin**, and **elemicin** are illustrations of catecholamine-like psychedelics. Their chemical structure is similar to the bodies' **endogenous** catecholamine neurotransmitters, norepinephrine and dopamine, and the **exogenous** substances, cocaine and amphetamine. These catecholamine agonists perform a complex dance between DA and 5HT, which confers the psychedelic properties.

Serotonin-like psychedelics are **LSD**, **DMT**, **psilocybin**, **psilocin**, **bufotenine**, **ololiuqui**, **ibogaine**, and **harmine**, whose psychedelic effects originate from the augmentation of serotonin neurotransmission.

Glutaminergic NMDA is **phencyclidine (PCP)** and structurally related compounds.

LSD

Lysergic acid diethylamide (lysergide), or LSD, is the most used psychedelic hallucinogenic in the United States. LSD is a potent synthetic serotonin-like hallucinogenic drug that is derived from the **ergot alkaloids**. It is a Schedule I drug, having no legitimate medicinal use and high potential for abuse. Slang names include acid, cubes, and purple haze. While LSD has a high potential for abuse, it has a very low dependency effect. LSD is swallowed, injected, dissolved and diluted in liquid, and sprayed or dripped on blotter paper or sugar cubes. The hallucinogen is prepared in the laboratory by chemical synthesis. LSD is rarely found in its pure form as it is poorly synthesized and usually contains other byproducts.

LSD is related structurally to **bufotenine**, **psilocybin**, **harmine**, and **ibogaine,** which bind and stimulate serotonin and dopamine receptors, increasing the neurotransmitter response.

LSD acts on both classes of serotonin receptors, blocking one while it stimulates the other. One serotonin group is stimulated while the other was found to be responsible for causing hallucinations. However, the research is still unclear since other drugs that increase serotonin levels in the brain do not seem to cause hallucinations. Additionally, LSD appears to increase glutamate release in the cerebral cortex. As an agonist on the 5HT receptors, consequences can be dramatic (Fantegrossi et al, 2008).

Onset of central nervous system effects is about 20 minutes, comprising of hypertension, dilated pupils, hyperthermia, tachycardia, and enhanced alertness. The psychoactive effects start in about 1–2 hours, with duration in the blood up to 72 hours and 24–72 hours in the urine. The LSD serotonergic and dopaminergic effects cause heightened perceptions; distortion of sensory and body perception; unpredictable moods; emotional swings; cognitive impairment; and hallucinations from wavering images, color patterns, and warping of size to more complex vivid visions and detailed scenes. Visions with closed eyes are a common feature as well as synesthesia, acute perception, emotional insights, and a sense of **ego disintegration**.

This mystification of the senses sometimes gives the user a profound understanding or enlightenment from their trip or becoming one with self or the universe. There is no current evidence of long-term effects or dangerous **physical reactions**; however, the **psychological consequences** can be dangerous and frightening. Changes in mood, time, and impulsive behavior can make the user paranoid and aggressive. LSD's effects can last from eight to ten hours, and, as the drug wears off, users often feel fatigued. **Bad trips** are common. Some LSD experiences lead to psychosis, toxic delirium, flashbacks, and violence. Treatment for a bad trip is supportive with a talkdown and medications. There is a higher incidence of **flashbacks** as the number of hallucinogenic experiences increase.

There is no general consensus that LSD is teratogenic and that it may cause possible reproductive detriment to humans and animal species by creating genetic damage.

Bufotenine administered orally is not hallucinogenic as it does not cross the blood brain barrier; however, 5-methoxyDMT, found in Bufo alvarius rather than Bufo marinus, is hallucinogenic when smoked. Bufotenine is highly toxic, and the reported psychedelic effects may be due to peripheral toxicity.

MDMA

The synthetic derivative designer drug, **MDMA** (methylenedioximetamphetamine), also goes by **Ecstasy,** Molly, love, and happy drug; it is a powerful stimulant and mood changer that accelerates body systems and modifies the perceptual field of the world. It is not a drug created in nature but synthesized in laboratories and garages, whose chemical structure is closely related to MDA and methamphetamine. It produces both stimulant and psychedelic effects by flooding the brain with the release of the neurotransmitter serotonin and by inhibiting the enzymes that degrade serotonin. MDMA is classified with no medical use, high abuse potential, and is illegal in the United States.

The increase in the usage and distribution of Ecstasy is partially due to the popularity of raves. Raves are underground parties that are open for nearly 12 hours. The rave party scene has often been compared to a religious or shamanistic ceremony. The DJ is the high priest of the ceremony, dancing is its meditation, and Ecstasy is its holy substance. The atmosphere of raves is designed to be favorable to enjoying the Ecstasy experience, which is a common venue for taking Ecstasy. Ecstasy, along with various drugs, is offered openly to the public. This is a familiar scene at raves, and security usually takes no steps in preventing it. Raves are known for having a blind-eye approach to drug taking and drug dealing.

Another contributor to the increase of MDMA users is that it is perceived as the "happy drug." MDMA stimulates the release of the neurotransmitter serotonin from brain neurons. This produces a rush of energy and is followed by a gradual sensation. MDMA can produce stimulant effects like enhanced sense of pleasure, self-confidence, and bouncing energy. Its psychedelic effects include feelings of peacefulness, acceptance, and empathy. Users claim that it causes euphoria; feelings of apprehension are eliminated and replaced by feelings of warmth and relaxation. Everyone is encouraged to think only "happy thoughts." At raves, everyone is neighborly and kindly offers water bottles, pacifiers, drugs, massages, and light shows to fellow ravers.

MDMA is a crystalline powder in tea or capsules. The effects stimulate the sympathetic nervous system also causing nausea, vomiting, diarrhea, and abdominal pain. Effects occur within minutes and last up to four to five hours. The serotonin neurotoxic effect increases impulsive and hostile behaviors along with depression. Ecstasy intensifies happiness; it also intensifies depression and fear. Its high will only last for a couple of hours, and the long-term health, memory, and psychological problems endure.

PCP

Phencyclidine (PCP) is known by many names, including angel dust, embalming fluid, killer weed, rocket fuel, wack, supergrass, and juice. It was approved for use as an investigational drug in clinical trials, but its medical use was short-lived due to hallucinations, delirium, dysphoria, confusion, psychosis, schizophrenia, and mania. By 1965, it was taken off the market, limiting the drug to veterinary use only as an injectable anesthetic, analgesic, and animal tranquilizer. In the late 1960s, it was introduced as a street drug for its ability to give users a sense of power, invincibility, and superhuman strength. Even after gaining a reputation as a drug with very unpleasant side effects, it grew to epidemic proportions during the 1970s.

Pharmacokinetics of PCP is a hallucinogenic drug that is available in various forms such as a white crystalline powder, tablets, crystals, and liquid. It can be snorted, smoked, ingested, or injected intravenously or subcutaneously. Well absorbed from all routes of administration, oral PCP takes effect in five minutes, lasts for about 6–8 hours, and can be found in the urine and blood for up to ten days.

Using PCP is referred to as getting wet or dusted. PCP's effects are dependent on the dosage and administration. Small doses produce numbness; intoxication; slurred speech; bloodshot eyes; **dissociative state** (feelings of detachment), feeling distant and estranged from surroundings; and loss of balance. Moderate doses will produce analgesia, anesthesia, a rise in blood pressure, feelings of strength, and a sense of invulnerability. High doses may lead to convulsions, coma, and death. Psychological effects include severe changes in body image, image distortion, and auditory hallucinations that can bring on severe mood swings, amnesia, paranoia, sometimes violent outbursts, and euphoria. Suicidal tendencies have also been reported.

The pharmacodynamics of PCP is as **noncompetitive NMDA receptor antagonist** and binding to **opioid and glutamate receptors** in the brain. These receptor antagonists induce **dissociative anesthesia** that are a class of hallucinogens, which distort the perceptions of sight and sound. They produce feelings of detachment from themselves and the environment, giving someone an "out-of-body"-like experience. It is believed that PCP has several sites of action in the central nervous system, all of which act together to result in anesthesia and analgesia. PCP inhibits dopamine, norepinephrine, and serotonin reuptake, and it increases dopamine and norepinephrine production. Some studies have found, like other NMDA receptor antagonists, phencyclidine can cause a kind of brain damage called **Olney's lesions,** which have been found in rats. All studies of Olney's lesions have only been performed on animals and may not apply to humans.

Chronic PCP use may cause physical dependency in users. It was at first thought that there was no withdrawal syndrome of PCP in humans until one group of users described a possible discontinuation syndrome; it happened within one day of discontinuing the use of PCP among outpatients who were daily users for at least three months. The syndrome included depression, anxiety, irritability, hypersomnia, increased appetite, poor memory, confused thoughts, and increased craving for PCP. However, it still remains unclear whether these symptoms represent a true drug withdrawal syndrome.

PCP can become addictive with its rewarding and reinforcing effects. Memory loss, depression, weight loss, and difficulty speaking and learning are some symptoms users can have. It has been found that young adults who have used PCP can have an interference with hormones that are used to help in development and normal growth. PCP intoxication has brought many users into emergency rooms, and, once there, they have become violent or suicidal, making them very dangerous. The general approach to detoxification and supportive care includes isolation in a quiet environment, supportive measures to prevent self-harming, maintenance of cardiorespiratory functions, and drug treatment for psychotic symptoms.

Removal of PCP can be aided by gastric lavage or drainage. Activated charcoal can be used for GI decontamination with patients that have recently orally taken PCP. The activated charcoal can be administered and repeated every four hours for several doses in order to absorb the PCP. Haloperidol or atypical antipsychotic, dopamine blockers have value in treating PCP-induced psychosis. When anxiety, agitation, and seizures are present, benzodiazepines are the common drug of choice for the situation. Due to some of PCP's long-lasting side effects that can induce or reveal psychopathologic symptoms, psychiatric hospitalization may be necessary for prolonged psychosis. Continuing outpatient therapy with possible use of tranquilizers may also be necessary after PCP intoxication.

Ketamine

Ketamine was originally developed as a **general anesthetic** in the early 60s (mass market by 1970). Ketamine was used in treating burn victims, alongside radiation therapy, and also for battlefield injuries during the Vietnam War. It was also preferred for use in children with hypersensitivity to anesthesia because it was less sedative. It was also used in some veterinary practices. Ketamine works by selectively interrupting association pathways to the brain, producing a sensory blockade. Ketamine causes **dissociation**, feelings of floating or separation or an out-of-body experience, and it can also raise blood pressure, whether by injection or ingestion; so it is contraindicated in patients with high or low blood pressure.

While ketamine usually has a wide margin of safety, it is, in particular, not used in some elderly patients because of its dizzying side effects. Ketamine is generally used for short surgical procedures though it can be used in longer procedures with extra dosing. There has been evidence reported that repeated ketamine users can develop a tolerance and/or dependence to the drug. The effects of ketamine are considered dose-dependent; lower doses produce varying results when compared to higher doses. Ketamine has a great deal in common with other drugs linked to dependence, such as opiates, stimulants, and alcohol.

The side effects of ketamine include anesthesia with sedation, aggressive behavior, hallucinations, amnesia, tachycardia, muscle weakness, dizziness, chest pain, anxiety, respiratory depression, and even **rhabdomyolysis**. These side effects can happen up to 24 hours after use. Some of these side effects are the reason why ketamine, with its LSD-like effect on the body, became an illicit drug. It is the **date rape drug** used in clubs or during raves. Ketamine can be very dangerous, and overdosing can be life threatening. Some of the slang terms for ketamine are Special K, Super K, Kit-Kat, Purple, or Mauve.

The FDA issued a warning about the illicit uses of ketamine in 1996, and it has been considered a C-III scheduled drug ever since. Though it is still on the market, it is rarely used and tightly restricted. Other examples of drugs in this class are PCP or DXM. Unfortunately, the way that ketamine is getting on the street is through diversion or theft of veterinarian offices, pharmacies, and pharmaceutical companies.

Psilocybin

Psilocybin, *Psilocybin Mexicana*, magic mushrooms or shrooms, is a serotonin-like psychedelic hallucinogen. It is a Schedule I, with an onset of effect in 30–60 minutes, duration of effect 5–6 hours. The serotonergic system affects mood and causes physical hallucinations of time, space, and perceptual alterations; many users feel a religious experience. Bad trips include the inability to concentrate, anxiety, panic, and paranoia.

Alpha Omega

"Twins, we were young teenagers, and she already had the inherent ability to cut hair, every kind of hair imaginable. Boys hair, girls hair, long hair, curly hair, she knew exactly how to maneuver scissors expertly around and between each strand until a perfectly coiffed style had emerged. This was even before training in a vocational college for hairstyling. I always wished I had her unwavering self-confidence and devil-may-care attitude. She was great in the kitchen, too, and surely didn't learn from Mom, who was a strictly meat-and-potatoes kind of cook catering to Dad's bland Irish taste buds. Yep, I always wanted to be more like my sister.

"Addiction really is an equal opportunity club. All are welcome no matter your status or social ranking. It arrives when you aren't looking; like some relatives, it stays too long. It wouldn't get me though. No, not me ...

"She jumped into the rough crowd right from the start. We transferred from the Midwest where we went to Catholic school. Yeah, we were good Catholic girls. Switching to public school in California was culture shock and a turning point, for sure. I gravitated to the shy kids who looked as scared and as lost as I was. My sister hit the ground running. She became popular with the football team and its cheerleaders, the stoners, too. Everyone loved her. She could be whoever you wanted her to be, as long as she was high.

"I was a well-kept secret for a long time. When word got out about me, they thought I must be the younger sister, certainly not her twin. I was invisible, or tried to be. I towed the line. It was easier, and why not? Not much to rebel against. We'd been brought up in a loving family, didn't want for much. Just do well in school and stay out of trouble. How hard could that be? Looking back, I see her demons came early, and they fought hard. Relentless they were. They've gotten stronger ... dangerous.

"Seems like a lifetime ago when we told each other secrets. Now our talk is reduced to please, please, dear sister, get help, again. Mom has the money and will pay anything for you to get better, again. Please, do it for your kids.

I know better though. Your kids can't get you sober. Mine tried to save me from the addictions that I swore would never catch me, silly me. It wasn't my choice. It wasn't hers.

"I live in a house. She lives on the street. I go to school. She goes to jail. I needed help; wanted help. She needs help; doesn't want help. She'll die on the streets. I'll die trying to save her. I know I can't save her. But she's my sister. She is my twin."—Anonymous

Critical Thinking

MORE STEPS --- THE PARADIGM

> "It is better to make many small steps in the right direction than to make one giant leap forward only to stumble backward."
>
> —Chinese Proverb

Sustainable energy is a popular catchall; however, what about humans' sustainable energy story? What about our core rituals and behaviors, motivated by devout processes of the learned stories that we tell ourselves? How can we have a positive impact and level of engagement in our slice of time and section of the neighborhood?

Overcoming inertia, apathy, inactivity, lethargy, inaction, sluggishness, and unwillingness requires the energy of motivation. Developing an energy plan to be open and receptive to tools and techniques that are individualized from person to person is the foundation of selecting what works for you. Identify rituals and emotions that cultivate positive change and work at discarding the rest. Perseverance, persistence, and practice are the devotion of time and energy.

Look at the meaning and purpose of the impulse, itch, yen, drive, stimulus, or urge. An integrative approach to seeing the old tapes, viewing our perception of life situations with a reverse, long, and wide lens will harvest the bigger picture.

Self-management and self-reflection are to be used to identify our underlying learned beliefs, critically evaluate these beliefs, and to reframe them with positive helpful views. Managing, handling, coping with thoughts, feelings, and behaviors that *float* through us with an inner reflective approach will heal past traumas and make positive change. Awareness brings reduction, then disintegration of pain and destructive behavioral patterns. To completely reframe adjusting how one's mind responds to the world through automatic responses, the blocked energy is released, and healing can take place and change happens.

SMART TOOLS

Point 1: Building and Maintaining Motivation
Point 2: Coping with Urges
Point 3: Managing Thoughts, Feelings, and Behaviors
Point 4: Living a Balanced Life

MOTIVATION TOOLS

1. Express empathy—be warm, respectful and accepting.
2. Develop discrepancy—amplify the difference between current behaviors and expressed personal goals and values.
3. Avoid argumentation—stay away from persuasion, confrontation, and argument.
4. Roll with resistance—redirect resistance with language; "it is really up to you."
5. Support self-efficacy—reframe "failures" as getting closer to the goal elicits hope.

Spiritus, the Latin word, means **to breathe**, the act of being **filled with air**, the **light** quality, which is **flexible and moves freely**. All origins are based on the teachings, grounded on ego deflation, honesty, moral inventory, restitution, working with others, and contrition. Core values practiced daily, in everyday behaviors, are to aspire and spiral with positive actions and feelings of well-being. It is, I am, or higher power, in alignment with self, highest level of integrity, source, universe, and oneness can resonate on an individual level.

WISH

HALLUCINOGENS

Overview of Psychoactive Drugs:

https://www.youtube.com/watch?v=icD3l5bhhKY

Psychoactive Drugs: Hallucinogens

https://www.youtube.com/watch?v=GUwV0gibLx8

LSD

What Does LSD Do to the Brain:

https://www.youtube.com/watch?v=LJbrLSU2Tk4

MDMA

Brain on MDMA:

https://www.youtube.com/watch?v=jEAr7ThsYew

PCP

Angel Dust:

https://www.youtube.com/watch?v=cMmzsER9xN8

KETAMINE

Ketamine Drug Education:

https://www.youtube.com/watch?v=l-8MepXYUig

Animation Effects of Ketamine:

https://www.youtube.com/watch?v=mV03EH3HVQ0

PSILOCYBIN

Brain on Shrooms

https://www.youtube.com/watch?v=F5kqThVON18

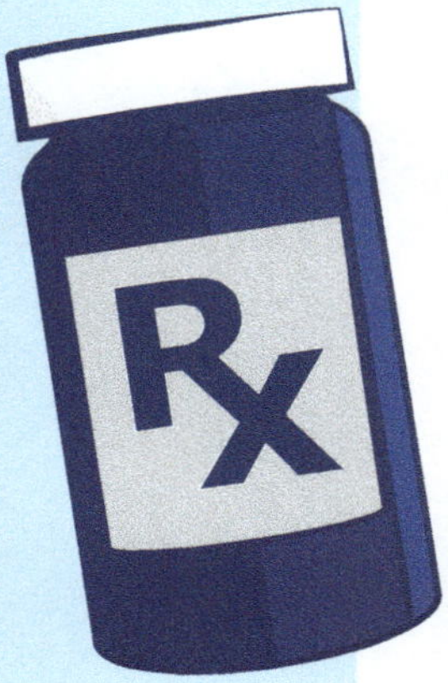

Drug Sandbox

IMPORTANT WORDS TO KNOW!

Psychomimetics
Psychedelics
Mescaline
Peyote
Psilocybin
Lysergic Acid Diethylamide (LSD)
Phencyclidine (PCP)
Dimethyltryptamine (DMT)
Methylenedioxyamphetamine (MDA)
2,5-Dimethoxy-4-Methylamphetamine (STP)
Acetylcholine Psychedelics
Catecholamine-like
Serotonin-like
Glutaminergic NMDA
Scopolamine
Hyoscyamine
Anticholinergic Syndrome
Ecstasy (MDMA)
DOM
MMDA
Myristin
Elemicin
Endogenous
Exogenous
Psilocin
Bufotenine
Ololiuqui,
Ergot Alkaloids
Harmine
Ibogaine
Ego Disintegration.
Physical Reactions
Psychological Consequences
Bad Trips
Flashbacks
Dissociation State

Noncompetitive NMDA Receptor Antagonist
Opioid and Glutamate Receptors
Dissociative Anesthesia
Olney's Lesions
General Anesthetic
Dissociation,
Rhabdomyolysis
Date Rape Drug

Community Connections

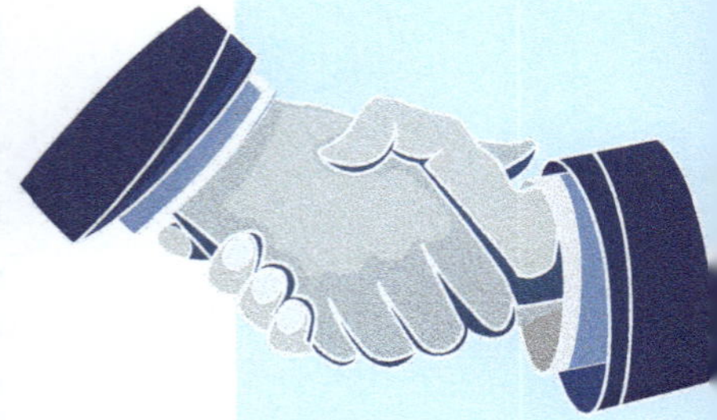

USE OF AYAHUASCA IN THE TREATMENT OF ADDICTION IN SOUTH AMERICA

In the past 40 years, several long-term research studies have examined the methods used by shamans to heal alcoholism and addiction with the Ayahuasca brew. Ayahuasca is an entheogen known to produce powerful hallucinations. An entheogen is a psychoactive substance used in a shamanic context predating written language. Ayahuasca induces an alteration of consciousness. It has been used safely in religious rituals for millennia in the Amazon Basin. This knowledge has been maintained orally by traditional healers. Ethnobotanist Richard Evans Schultes documented the plants involved in the preparation of Ayahuasca in Plants of the Gods. The Ayahuasca brew is a hallucinogenic beverage made from the decoction of the bark of a vine called Banisteriopsis caapi (which contains harmala alkaloids harmine, harmaline, and tetrahydroharmine) and the leaves of Psychotria viridis (which contain dimethyltryptamine or DMT, a potent hallucinogen enhancing the activation of the neurotransmitter serotonin).

Dimethyltryptamine is the main psychoactive ingredient in the Ayahuasca brew. Most often, the Ayahuasca brew is made with the bark of the Ayahuasca vine and the Chacruna plant, but sometimes other plants are added, such as Datura. It is always consumed in a specific healing ritual within the particular cultural context led by an experienced shaman. Acting as guide, the healer, or curandero, conducts the ceremony with his prayers and sacred songs. Shamanism is the most ancient form of spiritual practice associated with humans. It is an animist, nondogmatic form of religion that is polytheistic. Nature is considered sacred where everything is animated by spirits.

Extensive research on the therapeutic use of the psychotropic Ayahuasca has been conducted by Ralph Metzner, who is interested in its application in psychotherapy. In the Amazon Indian shamanistic worldview and cosmology, a symbolic death of the ego is followed by a rebirth. This is a central feature of the Ayahuasca experience, contributing to the healing process in addiction and recovery. Ayahuasca acts a catalyst. What appears essential is the ritual's structure and intention: "the conscious arranging of the set and setting for the purposes agreed upon by the shaman and the patient or initiate" (Meztner, p. 21). Occasionally, only the shaman ingests the plant medicine, and then he does extractions of negative entities on the patient suffering from addiction. He works on the energetic level or the spiritual level. When the patient actually drinks the brew, he or she takes it as a sacrament like a Catholic would consume the Eucharist (which could be considered a placebo entheogen in modern Christianity). The session is conducted in the dark of night. After an hour, the person ingesting the Ayahuasca brew will begin to have intense visions or powerful insights that may last up to six hours.

Benny Shanon in Antipodes of the Mind states, "Ayahuasca highly accentuates both sensory perceptions and affective response" (p. 311). The shaman creates an external stimulation with his icaros (sacred ceremony songs), whistling or using the sound of his rattle to put his patient in a trance state. Music becomes a conduit for the experience in the inner visual field, and it has a psychological impact that can be manipulated by the shaman to convey certain emotions. For Shanon, "music is unique in that it exhibits homomorphism under perception distortion or hallucination. Homomorphism is the property of mathematical mapping" (p. 351). By creating soothing sounds, the shaman encourages deep relaxation and concentration. This allows the participant to enter a state of trance characterized by a sense of heightened awareness during which the inner visual field is flooded with synesthetic perceptions even with the eyes closed. Kaleidoscopic visions with geometric designs are common.

Ayahuasca intake can make the drinker "shift from one cognitive experience to another" (p. 339). The songs and the whistling serve to structure the visions of the participants by calling in the different spirit helpers of the shaman. Surrendering to a higher power energetically takes place. Images appear in the mind's eye, communicating like the mysterious language of dreams. Ayahuasca sensitizes perception, including spiritual, life-changing insights.

The addicted patient, having taken Ayahuasca, might also vomit violently or purge through a bowel movement. This is also a regular occurrence in Peyote ceremonies. In Ayahuasca rituals, this purging reaction is the result of high serotonin levels in the intestines: it is considered a powerful detoxification process on all levels (physical, psychological, mental, and spiritual). Native American Indians call this humbling process "getting well." For this reason, these sacred entheogens are not used recreationally because they are too powerful and can be very frightening. Furthermore, they do require the assistance of a shaman who is very familiar with the psychic processes in order to enter the unchartered territories of the magical visions brought on by the medicine songs.

In Brazil, two major churches were founded in the 1950s that involved the drinking of Yage or Ayahuasca. These syncretic religious movements are the Santo Daime Church and Uniao do Vegetal. These organizations now exist in North America and in Europe. These groups have thousands of members and have participated in long-term research to study the effect of these plants on addiction (Grob et al. 1996). Metzner mentions that "the Brazilian Hoasca Project reported a marked decline in alcoholism and drug addiction among church members" (p. 250). These same scientists, Grob from UCLA and Dobkin de Rios from UC Irvine, worked on the Hoasca Project in 1996, conducting another empirical study doing a drug substitution with entheogens (Ayahuasca, Ibogaine, and Peyote) while adding the concept of redemption in the religious worldwide context (Data from Africa, Brazil, Peru, USA). "The redemptive model combined with the proper use of one psychoactive substance within a spiritual or clinical context helps to free an individual from the adverse effects of [his or her] addiction to another substance and thus restores [him or her] as functioning members of [his or her] community or group" (Dobkin de Rios 2002).

In Peru, the Takiwasi Program was started by a French doctor named Jacques Mabit in 1992. This center for the rehabilitation of drug addicts and for research of traditional medicine is located in Tarapoto. Patients with cocaine addiction are treated using Ayahuasca and other native plants from the Amazon with the help of local shamans and a team of Peruvian psychologists. This experimental center is a nonprofit organization and has been supported for decades by the French Government, the E.E.C, and the U.N. in order to develop an alternative therapy in the treatment of drug addictions. Takiwasi receives outpatients in recovery and outside researchers interested in scientific study. Although it is a small operation, Takiwasi has shown a high rate of 60% success in treating addicts as opposed to 10% in the USA, on average, in rehabilitation centers across the nation. The very high success rate and relatively low cost are a positive aspect; however, Ayahuasca is not available or legal in the USA.

In Holland, the UK, and Portugal, ibogaine has been used successfully to help heroin addiction (Alper, 1999). A potent root from Africa, ibogaine promotes long-term abstinence from addictive substances in a short period, with none of the usual side effects, such as the painful physical withdrawal symptoms. In the USA, Arapaho Indian participants in Peyote ceremonies within the Native American Church have been studied to examine their ability to heal themselves from alcoholism (Dombrowe, 2005).

As more research on the healing role of Ayahuasca in the treatment of addictions develops, a bridge is created between science and ancient spiritual practices using sacred entheogen plants. The Takiwasi Program and the Hoasca Project demonstrate an effort of cooperation between scientific medical teams and traditional ways of healing by shamans in order to improve the collective knowledge about ways to approach alternative treatments for addiction. Hopefully, these exchanges will bring more consciousness about Ayahuasca and the conservation of the Amazon. Additionally, they will inspire a tolerant respect for plant shamanism.

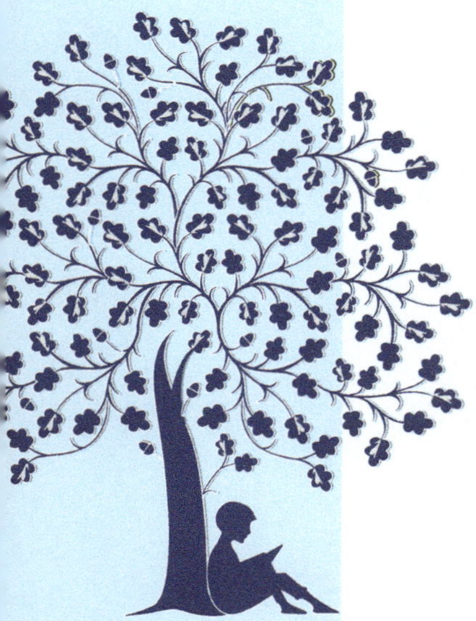

End Of Chapter Review Questions

Select the letter that matches the following words with their appropriate meanings (the letters may be used more than once):

1. PCP
2. LSD
3. Scopolamine
4. Psilocybin
5. Hyoscyamine
6. Ecstasy
7. Mescaline
8. Ketamine

a. Catecholamine-like psychedelic
b. Date Rape Drug
c. Serotonin-like psychedelic
d. Anticholinergic psychedelic
e. Glutaminergic NMDA

Multiple Choices: Select the best answer from the choices given:

9. ____________ causes dissociation, floating, or separation, an out-of-body experience; also known as the date rape drug.
    a. Diazepam
    b. Chlordiazepoxide
    c. Alprazolam
    d. Clonazepam
    e. Ketamine

10. Anticholinergic syndrome symptoms include:
    a. Hot flashes, hot as a hare
    b. Visual accommodation impairment, blind as a bat
    c. Reduced secretions, dry as a bone
    d. Peripheral vasodilation, red as a beet
    e. Psychosis, mad as a hen
    f. All of the above

11. LSD derives from:
    a. Elemicin
    b. Ergot alkaloids
    c. Methadone
    d. Morphine
    e. Mushrooms

12. Bad trips and flashbacks are common with which serotonin-like psychedelic?
    a. LSD
    b. PCP
    c. DOM
    d. DMT
    e. MMDA

13. A dissociation state and induced dissociative anesthesia most commonly occurs from ________ binding to opioid and glutamate receptors.
    a. LSD
    b. PCP
    c. DOM
    d. DMT
    e. MMDA

14. Which substance can cause **rhabdomyolysis?**
    a. LSD
    b. PCP
    c. Ketamine
    d. Mescaline
    e. Scopolamine

15. *Spiritus*, the Latin word, means:
    a. To breathe
    b. The act of being filled with air
    c. A light quality
    d. Flexible and moves freely
    e. All of the above

16. Olney's lesions, a type of brain damage, may be associated with:
    a. LSD
    b. PCP
    c. DOM
    d. DMT
    e. MMDA

17. Bufotenine is a:
    a. Acetylcholine psychedelic
    b. Catecholamine-like psychedelic
    c. Serotonin-like psychedelic
    d. Glutaminergic NMDA psychoactive drug.

18. Which of the following statements regarding bufotenine is incorrect?
    a. It is not a hallucinogen.
    b. It does not cross the blood brain barrier.
    c. It is administered orally.
    d. It is not toxic.

19. Which of the following statements regarding Ayahuasca is correct?
    a. It is used by shamans to heal alcoholism and addiction.
    b. It is an entheogen known to produce powerful hallucinations.
    c. It induces an alteration of consciousness.

d. It has been used safely in religious rituals for millennia in the Amazon Basin.
e. All of the above are correct.

20. Which of the following statements regarding the steps to sustainable human energy is most correct?
    a. Inertia must be overcome.
    b. Look at the meaning.
    c. Look at the bigger picture.
    d. Involves self-management and self-reflection.
    e. All of the above are steps and correct.

Applications: Assessment of Usage and Relevance

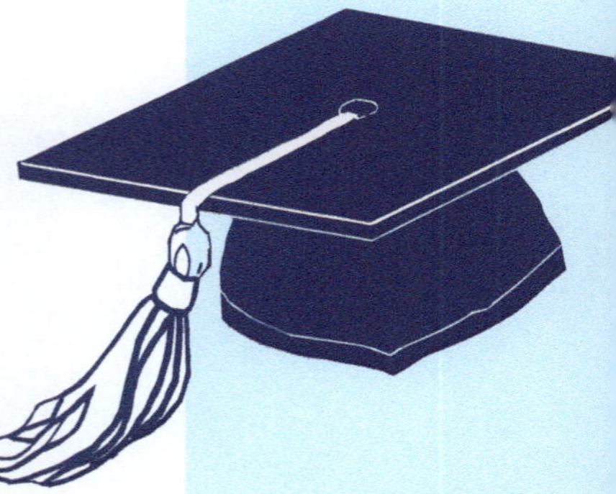

1. Describe, with examples, the families of psychedelics and hallucinogens.
2. Describe, with examples, the three ways acetylcholine psychedelics act.
3. Tell one interesting story about the history of use of psychedelic drugs.
4. What are designer drugs? How do they act?
5. What are the catecholamine-like psychedelics? Where do they act? Outline their families; use examples.

KEY

1. E	6. A	11. B	16. B
2. C	7. A	12. A	17. C
3. D	8. B	13. B	18. D
4. C	9. E	14. C	19. E
5. D	10. F	15. E	20. E

REFERENCES

Aaronson, Bernard, and Osmond, Humphry. Psychedelics: the use and implications of hallucinogenic drugs. 1970. New York, N.Y: Anchor Books/ Doubleday Inc.

Dishotsky et al. LSD and genetic damage. 1971. Science.172: 431–440.

Fantegrossi, William et al. The behavioral pharmacology of Hallucinogens. Biochem Pharmacol. 2008. 75(1): 17–33. Doi: 10-1016/j.

Kast, E. Pain and LSD-25: a theory of attenuation of anticipation. In Solomon, D. LSd: the Consciousness Expanding drug. 1964a. New York: Putnam.

Levinthal, Charles. Drugs, behavior and modern society. (2008). Boston: Allyn & Bacon Inc.

McGlothlin, William et al,. Effect of LSD on human pregnancy. 1970. JAMA. 212.9:1483–1487.

Zec, Natasa et al. Developmental changes in Lysergic acid diethylamide. Journal of Neuropathology and Experimental Neurology. 1996. 55.1: 114–126.

Brenner, Stephan. PCP Toxicity. 2014.

http://emedicine.medscape.com/article/1010821-overview.

Malenka, R. C., Nestler, E. J., and Hyman S. "Chapter 15: Reinforcement and Addictive Disorders." 2009.

Burns, R. S., Lerner, S., Corrado, R. Phencyclidine States of Acute Intoxication and Fatalities. 1975.

http://www.drugs.com/illicit/pcp.html.

Keltner, N., and Folks, D., Psycotropic Drugs, 4th Edition, Elsevier Mosby, 2005.

http://www.cesar.umd.edu/cesar/drugs/ketamine.asp.

http://www.nhtsa.gov/people/injury/research/job185drugs/ketamine.htm.

Portrayal Paradigm

Forcehimes, A., and Tonigan, J. Self-efficacy as a factor in abstinence from alcohol/other drug abuse: A meta-analysis. Alcoholism Treatment Quarterly. 2008:26(4):480–489.

Groh, D. R., Jason L., and Keys, C. Clin Psychol Rev. 2008 Mar; 28(3):430–50.

Schwartz, Tony. Managing your Energy. Harvard Business Review. October 2007. hbr.org.

Treatment of Drug Abuse and Addiction—Part III, The Harvard Mental Health Letter, Volume 12, Number 4, October 1995, page 3.

Tonigan, J., Toscova, R., and Miller, W. J. Stud Alcohol. 1996 Jan; 57(1):65–72.

Robinson, E. A. R., Krentzman, A. R., Webb, J. R., and Brower, K. J. (2011). Six-Month Changes in Spirituality and Religiousness in Alcoholics Predict Drinking Outcomes at Nine Months. Journal of Studies on Alcohol and Drugs, 72(4), 660–668.

http://www.rapidresolutiontherapy.com/.

Corey, S., Corey, M., Corey, G., and Corey, C. (2012). Group process and practice, 9th edition. Brooks/Cole Cengage Learning Publications, 128–129.

Substance Abuse and Mental Health Services Administration (2014). Substance abuse treatment: group therapy—a treatment improvement protocol, TIP 41. Department of Health and Human Services, Washington, D.C., 16–17.

SMART Recovery, Self-Management And Recovery Training (2015). http://www.smartrecovery.org/.

"SMART —Self Management for Addiction Recovery."Self Help Addiction Recovery. Web. 19 Sept. 2015. http://www.smartrecovery.org/.

"How Smart Is Smart Recovery? | The Fix" The Fix. Web. 19 Sept. 2015. http://www.thefix.com/content/how-smart-smart-recovery.

"The Emergence and Controversy of SMART Recovery." Sober Nation. Web. 19 Sept. 2015. http://www.sobernation.com/the-emergence-and-controversy-of-smart-recovery/.

"Why SMART Recovery Is an Increasingly Important Alternative to AA—Substance.com." Substancecom. 30 June 2014. Web. 19 Sept. 2015. http://www.substance.com/why-smart-recovery-is-an-increasingly-important-alternative-to-aa/8223/.

Edelman, D. "Disadvantages of Motivational Interviewing Model." http://www.ehow.com/list_6184181_disadvantages-motivational-interviewing-model.html.

Holleran Steiker, L. K., Motivational Interviewing and Addiction: An Interview With Melinda Hohman, Journal of Social Work Practice in the Addictions, Vol. 9, 2009.

Miller, W. R., and Rollnick, S, Motivational interviewing: Preparing people for change. 2nd ed. New York: Guilford Press; 2002.

Miller, W. R. , and Rose, G. S. Toward a Theory of Motivational Interviewing, Sept. 1, 2010. http://www.ncbi.nlm.nih.gov/pmc/articles/PMC2759607/#R52.

Slate, S., "The Tragedy of Motivational Interviewing," Feb. 18, 2011. http://www.the-cleanslate.org/the-tragedy-of-motivational-interviewing/.

Van Wormer, K., and Davis, D. R., Addiction Treatment: A strengths Perspective, 3rd Edition, Brooks/Cole, 2013.

Community Connections

Alper, K. 2000. Treatment of acute opioid withdrawal with Ibogaine. The American Journal on Addictions. Vol 8. Summer 1999. p. 234–242.

Dobkin de Rios, M. 1994. Hallucinogens and Redemption. Journal of Psychoactive Drugs. Vol 34.

Dombrowe, C. 2005. CIIS, US. Touched by Spirit: A heuristic study of healing experiences in Peyote ceremonies. Dissertation Abstracts International. Vol 66 (5-B).

Grob, C. S., and M. Dobkin de Rios. Adolescent drug use in cross cultural perspective. Journal of Drug issues Vol 22. p121–38. 1992.

Mabit, J. 1988. Ayahuasca Hallucinations among Healers in the Peruvian Upper Amazon. Newsletter of the Multidisciplinary Association for Psychedelic Studies. Vol. 6, No. 3, 1996.

Meztner, Ralph. 2006. Ayahuasca, Sacred Vine of Spirits. Park Street Press, Vermont.

Shanon, Benny. The Antipodes of the Mind. 2002. Oxford University Press, New York.

Schultes, R. 1967. The place of Ethnobotany in the Ethno pharmacologic search for psychoactive drugs. Ethno pharmacologic search for psychoactive drugs, ed. D. Hefron.

CHAPTER EIGHT

NEUROMODULATORS

Chapter Objectives

1. Differentiate between typical and atypical antipsychotic medications.
2. Interpret objective and subjective symptoms of psychiatric disorders.
3. Differentiate among the types of antidepressant medication classifications.
4. Describe bipolar disorder and its management.
5. Identify the risks and benefits associated with the utilization of anabolic steroids and human growth hormone.

Positive Affirmations

> "Keep away from people who try to belittle your ambition. Small people always do that, but the really great make you feel that you, too, can become great."
>
> —Mark Twain

NEUROMODULATORS

Neuromodulators are a subset of neurotransmitters. They are substances released by a neuron, which transmits information to other neurons, altering their activities. Neuromodulators alter nerve impulse transmission. They are biologically active substances; for example, endorphins and substance P act locally on other neurons or at a distance, increasing or decreasing the intensity of effect of neurotransmitters; however, they themselves do not initiate electrical depolarization.

Neuromodulation is the process by which nervous activity is regulated as a way of controlling the physiological levels of several classes of neurotransmitters. Unlike neurotransmitters, the release of neuromodulators occurs in a diffuse manner through volume transmission. This means that the entire neural tissue may be subject to the neuromodulator's action upon exposure.

This, in turn, can fine-tune the neural circuitry of an entire brain region, not just that of an individual neuron. This is in contrast with the release of a neurotransmitter, which occurs at a specific synapse during direct synaptic transmission. Furthermore, neuromodulators and neurotransmitters act on different types of neuroreceptors. Neurotransmitters target fast-acting ionic neuroreceptors that convey electrochemical signals into the target neuron; neuromodulators target the slower G-protein neuroreceptors. Neuromodulation, unlike that of neurotransmission, does not necessarily carry excitation or inhibition from one neuron to another. Instead, it alters the cellular or synaptic properties of certain neurons so that neurotransmission between them is changed.

This is a physiological process that a given neuron uses to regulate diverse populations of neurons. It is in contrast to classical synaptic transmission, in which one presynaptic neuron directly influences a single postsynaptic partner. Neuromodulators secreted by a small group of neurons diffuse through large areas of the nervous system, affecting multiple neurons. Major neuromodulator systems in the central nervous system affect dopamine, serotonin, acetylcholine, histamine, and norepinephrine neurotransmitters.

Neuromodulators pass a significant amount of time in the cerebrospinal fluid (CSF), influencing or modulating the activity of several other neurons in the brain. For this reason, some neurotransmitters are also considered to be neuromodulators, such as serotonin and acetylcholine. Thereby, some neurotransmitters become agents of change in the central nervous system, potentially allowing for plasticity!

Antipsychotics

Antipsychotics, also known as neuroleptics or major tranquilizers, are a class of psychiatric medication primarily used to manage psychosis, including delusions, hallucinations, or disordered thought. They are integral in the treatment of schizophrenia and bipolar disorder and have been found useful in the management of nonpsychotic disorders. First-generation antipsychotics, known as typical antipsychotics, include haloperidol (Haldol), perphenazine (Trilafon), **and** chlorpromazine (Thorazine). First generation antipsychotics can cause tardive dyskinesia, the involuntary movement of the face, tongue, jaw, neck, and extremities, as well as pseudo-Parkinson's-like symptoms. They work well on the management of positive symptoms of schizophrenia and delirium in the elderly but not on negative symptoms.

Second-generation drugs, known as atypical antipsychotics, include aripiprazole (Abilify), olanzapine (Zyprexa), quetiapine (Seroquel), Ziprasidone (Geodon), **and** risperidone (Risperdal). They are generally preferred because they pose a lower risk of serious side effects. Atypical antipsychotics act on multiple receptor types, including dopamine and serotonin, with higher selectivity for dopamine receptors. Atypical antipsychotics generally have lower risk of motor side effects. They are associated with significant weight gain, hyperglycemia, and elevated lipids and prolactin. A trademark of atypical antipsychotics is the near absence of extrapyramidal side effects. Clozapine (Clozaril) is used in treatment-resistant schizophrenia. It lowers white blood cell count, causing agranulocytosis, a life-threatening condition. Lithium is a mineral that has no psychotropic effect in normal people. It is useful in the treatment of bipolar disorder and is associated with a reduction of suicides.

Subjective and objective symptoms of psychiatric mental disorders for people who suffer from them, such as schizophrenics, may include auditory distortions (hearing voices); distortions of thinking; inability to think and reason clearly; paranoia (others can hear their thoughts or are trying to harm them or they are the President of the United States or some other famous person); visual distortions; hallucinations; delusions; confusion; and disorganized speech. They may get excited or angry for no apparent reason or spend a lot of time by themselves or in bed, sleeping during the day and staying awake at night. They may neglect their appearance, not bathe or change clothes, and may be hard to talk to, barely speaking or saying things that make no sense. These are positive symptoms.

Negative symptoms of schizophrenia are limited speech and emotional expression, lack of motivation, flat affect, and apathy. The schizophrenic patient is unable to relate to reality. It is a serious disability with a high incidence of suicides. Contributing factors are genetic, early environmental factors (fetal exposure to infection or malnutrition), drug abuse (cannabis, amphetamine, cocaine), and social stressors such as extreme poverty. Low glutamate levels are believed to contribute to the schizophrenic symptoms. Schizophrenics often are unaware initially that their condition is an illness.

These behaviors are mediated by higher than normal levels of dopamine and an imbalance of other neurotransmitters. Antipsychotic drugs' mechanism of action appears to be postsynaptic blockade of dopaminergic receptors, thereby, interfering with dopaminergic transmission and dampening the neurotransmitters and symptoms. These dopamine receptor antagonists are responsible for the antipsychotic action and cause very little tolerance and no physical dependence with an absence of addiction potential. Some medications block acetylcholine, serotonin, norepinephrine, and histamine. By blocking dopamine function in the brain, the psychotic symptoms are reduced by typical antipsychotic medication. The atypical antipsychotic medications do affect serotonin function and have less of a dopamine blocking effect. Abnormally low levels of the neurotransmitter glutamate were found in the brains of deceased schizophrenic patients, leading to the discovery of glutamate-blocking drugs like ketamine.

Both generations of medication block receptors in the brain's dopamine pathways. Atypical antipsychotics act on serotonin receptors, as well. Antipsychotics are more effective than placebo in treating symptoms of psychosis; however, some people do not respond fully or even partly to treatment. This therapeutic classification is associated with significant side effects, most notably movement disorders and weight gain.

Side effect profile includes muscle stiffness, tremor, dry mouth, sedation, drowsiness, rapid heartbeat, dizziness when changing position, abnormal movements, and anticholinergic effects. Neuroleptic malignant syndrome and tardive dyskinesia are rare but serious side effects. Many lessen or disappear after the first few weeks of treatment. The long-term outcome of psychotic episodes is dependent upon consistent pharmacological treatment. These medications do not cure the illness; however, they can minimize the symptoms, shorten the course of an episode, and improve the quality of life.

Psychiatric Indications

- Schizophrenia
- Manic episodes
- Bipolar
- OCD
- Post-traumatic stress disorder
- Tourette's syndrome
- Dementia
- Autism

Nonpsychiatric Indications

- Antiemetic, anesthesia

Acute Extrapyramidal Effects

- Akathisia: anxious pacing, rocking, fiddling, motor restlessness
- Dystonia: spasms and posturing, involuntary muscle contractions
- Pseudo-parkinsonism
- Tardive dyskinesia late onset > 6 months, involuntary movement limbs, trunk, and lips

Anticholinergic Side Effects

- Dry mouth
- Blurred vision
- Rapid heart rate (tachycardia)
- Urine retention
- Constipation
- Confusion and memory impairment

Minimize Antipsychotic Medications Side Effects with:

- Dimenhydrinate
- Benztropine
- Diphenhydramine
- Trihexyphenidyl
- Benzodiazepines

Antidepressants

"Depression is a mood disorder that causes a persistent feeling of sadness and loss of interest; also called major depressive disorder or clinical depression" (Mayo Clinic). There are many types of antidepressant medications used to treat depression on the market in the United States.

What is Depression?

- Depressed mood
- Feelings of guilt
- Impaired concentration
- Loss of interest
- Fatigue
- Sleep and weight changes
- Suicidal thoughts

They influence four major modulatory networks in the brain: serotonin, dopamine, norepinephrine, and acetylcholine. All seek to utilize the natural functioning chemical messages in the central nervous system. By manipulating this natural machinery, medications serve to enhance the effects of neurotransmitter release and availability by slowing neurotransmitter metabolism, preventing neurotransmitter reuptake, and using selective receptor antagonism. Realigning chemical imbalances of neurotransmitters in the brain will change mood and behavior. A wide range of conditions are indicated for antidepressant medications. They include social anxiety disorder, anxiety disorders, dysthymia, major depressive disorder, obsessive-compulsive disorder, panic disorder, post-traumatic stress disorder, premenstrual dysphoric disorder (PMDD), enuresis, chronic pain, and depression.

Selective serotonin reuptake inhibitors (SSRIs) have become the drug of choice in the treatment of depression, anxiety, avoidance behavior, and intrusive recollections. While they are not more effective than previous therapeutic classifications, they have a faster onset of action with less side effects and increased safety. SSRIs are also used to treat panic disorders, obsessive-compulsive disorders, obesity, and alcoholism. The FDA has approved paroxetine (Paxil) and sertraline (Zoloft) for the treatment of post-traumatic stress disorder (PTSD).

Neuroscientists have discovered a strong link between depression and low serotonin levels. By increasing serotonin levels in the brain, these signs will abate. SSRIs selectively block the reuptake of serotonin (5-HT), preventing the recycling by the synapse, thereby, increasing the serotonin concentration and duration in the synaptic cleft. SSRIs do not affect norepinephrine (NE), histamine, or acetylcholine (ACH); therefore, they do not produce sedation or cardiovascular and anticholinergic effects.

SSRI examples include fluoxetine (Prozac®), sertraline (Zoloft®), paroxetine (Paxil®), citalopram (Celexa), escitalopram (Lexapro), and fluvoxamine (Luvox). Venlafaxine (Effexor®), is a dual action product that inhibits both serotonin and norepinephrine pathways. Duloxetine (Cymbalta) is also a serotonin norepinephrine reuptake inhibitor (SNRI). SNRIs block the reuptake of both 5-HT and NE. Another agent, Mirtazapine (Remeron®), increases NE and 5-HT transmission by blocking alpha-2 auto-receptors for monoamines and blocking serotonin 2 and 3 receptors. It has been shown to be superior to other SSRIs in patients with depression associated with severe insomnia and anxiety.

Side effects may appear within 24 hours of the first dose; however, therapeutic effect can take up to 6–8 weeks. SSRIs have a low potential for overdose. Treatment is symptomatic and supportive.

Side effects may include restlessness, nervousness, anxiety, agitation, sweating, dry mouth, tachycardia, anorexia, increased appetite, weight gain, movement disorders, nausea, diarrhea, headache, insomnia, drowsiness, and sexual dysfunction. A potentially life-threatening effect of Serotonin syndrome can occur when SSRIs are combined with other serotonin agonists or drugs that interfere with the metabolism of 5-HT. This includes natural products, such as the Valerian root. Resolution of syndrome occurs within 48 hours of cessation of substance. Abruptly discontinuing an SSRI can cause withdrawal symptoms that persist for several weeks. A gradual decreasing tapering dose is recommended.

Serotonin Syndrome

- Severe agitation
- Disorientation and confusion
- Ataxia, increased reflexes
- Muscle spasms
- Fever, shivering, chills, diarrhea
- Elevated blood pressure and heart rate

Withdrawal Effects from SSRIs

- Dizziness
- Ataxia

- Nausea and vomiting
- Diarrhea
- Fatigue and chills
- Sensory disturbances
- Insomnia
- Vivid dreams
- Increased anxiety, agitation, and irritability

All SSRIs (except paroxetine) are classified as pregnancy Category C as they may not be safe for use during pregnancy. Category C in animal reproduction studies has shown adverse effects on the fetus. There are no adequate and well-controlled studies in humans; however, the potential benefits must warrant use of the drug in pregnant women despite potential risks. Paroxetine (Paxil, Paxil CR) is a Category D medication. Paroxetine may cause heart defects or serious, life-threatening lung problems in newborn babies whose mothers take the medication during pregnancy. SSRI use during pregnancy has been linked to autism and developmental delays in males.

Tricyclic antidepressants (TCAs) are another class of antidepressant drugs. Along with inhibiting serotonin reuptake, TCAs also inhibit the reuptake of norepinephrine, another neurotransmitter involved in mood elevation. By blocking reuptake pumps on the serotonergic and norepinephrinergic synapses, the concentrations of these neurotransmitters are maintained in the synaptic cleft. TCAs, however, are not as selective as SSRIs and have also exhibited interactions with histamine and acetylcholine. Due to their broader spectrum, antidepressants of this class are typically associated with more side effects.

Tricyclic antidepressants (TCA) inhibit the reuptake of neurotransmitters and block the effects of Ach, histamine, and alpha-adrenergic receptors. This is a leading factor in their side effect profile.

- Histamine blockade leads to sedation, fatigue.
- Ach blockade leads to the anticholinergic side effects of dry mouth, constipation, urinary retention, dizziness, confusion, blurred vision, and impaired memory.
- Alpha-1 blockade with the NE reuptake-blocking effect leads to cardiovascular side effects, including orthostatic hypotension, tachycardia, and arrhythmias that may cause cardiac arrest.

Pharmacodynamics of TCAs includes blockade of presynaptic receptors and transporters for serotonin, dopamine, and norepinephrine as well as blockade of different numbers of postsynaptic receptors for acetylcholine and histamine. The main antihistamine effect is drowsiness. These multiple actions of TCAs may be an advantage, for example, promoting sleep.

While the tricyclics are effective in blocking reuptake of NE and 5-HT, they also have anticholinergic activity which causes the side effects of sedation, weight gain, hypotension, blurred vision, dry mouth, constipation, urinary retention, confusion, delirium, ataxia, and tachycardia. Additional effects include dizziness, sexual dysfunction, impaired memory or cognitive function, and worsening of heart disease, seizures, and schizophrenia. While this drug is effective in treating depression, due to the side effects generated, SSRIs are highly recommended.

Imipramine (Tofranil®) was discovered as a modification of a phenothiazine antipsychotic. It is metabolized to desipramine which inhibits the reuptake of NE or 5-HT at the presynaptic neuron. The medication has a similar side effect profile which includes impairment of mental or physical abilities, seizures, and respiratory difficulties.

Amitriptyline (Elavil®) has higher sedative and anticholinergic effects and affects serotonin more than imipramine. This agent is often prescribed.

Clomipramine (Anafranil®) has the highest serotonin effect of the TCAs, with little anticholinergic or sedative action.

Desipramine (Norpramin®) is the active metabolite of imipramine with less anticholinergic effects. It increases concentrations of norepinephrine (NE) by inhibiting the reuptake at the presynaptic neuronal membrane. It is used cautiously in patients with cardiovascular disease, seizure disorders, urinary retention, glaucoma, hyperthyroidism, and with patient's receiving thyroid replacement. Desipramine may impair mental and physical abilities. Trimipramine (Surmontil®), protryptyline (Vivactil®), nortriptyline (Aventil®), and doxepin (Sinequan®) have suggestive trade names. All TCAs are toxic to the heart at high doses and are effective agents of suicide. This fact has fueled the search for other antidepressants.

Second-generation (Atypical Antidepressants) Non-SSRIs:

- Maprotiline (Ludiomil®) is based on the TCA molecule. May cause seizures and accumulates to toxic levels; more lethal than TCAs; blocks reuptake of NE.
- Amoxapine (Asendin®) blocks reuptake of NE and DA and may produce Parkinsonism.
- Bupropion (Wellbutrin®) selectively blocks DA uptake but is not reinforcing and may work when other antidepressants do not. Also used for AD/HD, nicotine craving (Zyban®).

Monoamine oxidase (MAO) inhibitors have demonstrated positive effects on mood, severe anxiety, and eating disorders. MAO inhibitors block the MAO enzyme that metabolizes monoamine neurotransmitters, norepinephrine, dopamine, and serotonin, increasing the amount available for release as well as the action at the receptor sites. For example, once serotonergic synapses have released serotonin into the synaptic cleft, it will diffuse across the space between the neurons, transiently bind to the serotonergic receptor on the postsynaptic membrane, and then be released back into the synaptic cleft. The neurotransmitter will then be removed from the synapse via reuptake by the serotonergic receptors on the presynaptic membrane or through degradation by monoamine oxidase. MAOIs, as their name implies, block the ability of monoamine oxidase to bind with monoamine neurotransmitters such as dopamine or serotonin. This increases the concentration and action of these neurotransmitters to continue to bind receptors on the postsynaptic cleft, initiating cellular responses that result in elevated moods.

MAOIs are used for treatment-resistant depression after SSRIs and/or TCAs have been shown to be ineffective. They have numerous side effects. The combination of SSRI and MAOI can lead to the potentially lethal serotonin syndrome. Rapid death from hyperthermia has also been reported. There needs to be a two-week washout interval between discontinuation of one treatment and initiation of another.

Side effects include cardiovascular increases in blood pressure and heart rate, anxiety, orthostasis, insomnia, sexual dysfunction, and weight gain. Any substance that elevates norepinephrine will have a much greater effect than normal. Therefore, nasal sprays, cold medications, amphetamines, and cocaine can produce dangerous side effects. Food products rich in tyramine; fermented, pickled foods; cheese; yogurt; sour cream; chocolate; avocados; soy sauce; tea; coffee; and alcohol must be avoided when taking this agent due to eliciting cardiovascular crisis. This class of antidepressants must be closely monitored when prescribed. Phenelzine (Nardil), selegiline (Deprenyl), tranylcypromine (Parnate), and isocarboxazid (Marplan) are currently available.

St. John's wort **and** SAM-e are considered natural remedies. They are first-line therapy in many European countries; however, they are not eagerly accepted by the clinical community in the United States. In the treatment of mild to moderate depression, St. John's wort has been found to be superior to placebo. It is also used for anxiety and weight gain. The agent has multiple drug interactions due to its effect on the liver enzyme system cytochrome P450. Side effects include photosensitivity, fatigue, dizziness, dry mouth, and paradoxical anxiety. SAM-e, S-adenosylmethionine, occurs naturally in the body and is involved in the synthesis of dopamine, serotonin, and other neurotransmitters. Various double-blind studies have shown SAM-e to be superior to placebo for depression. SAM-e is associated with manic symptoms, and there is limited drug interaction information. The evidence does not support an advantage of either agent in comparison to prescription antidepressants.

From a pharmacological perspective, antidepressant medications are of important use. Caution must be used in their administration as various complications of drugs interactions and/or tolerability may ensue. Antidepressant medication, used under the guidance of a mental health professional, may relieve some depression symptoms and improve the patient's quality of life.

In development are third generation antidepressants. Ketamine is a dissociative anesthetic that can be a substance of abuse. Ketamine has shown rapid reduction of depression symptoms within hours for 65 to 70 percent of treatment-resistant patients. Further study is needed.

Behavior Modifiers

—*Bipolar Disorder*

Bipolar disorder was previously known as manic depression, characterized by fluxing events of mania and depression. Classic symptoms include inflated self-esteem, talkativeness, decreased need for sleep, excessive activity, racing thoughts, and impairment of function. Hypomania is similar, with less harsh and incapacitating mood. The mood spectrum breadth ranges from severe depression to mild/moderate depression to normal to hypomania to mania or mixed mania.

Mood stabilizing agents and behavior modifiers include lithium (Eskalith, Lithobid); neuromodulators anticonvulsants, carbamazepine (Tegretol), oxcarbazepine (Trileptal), lamotrigine (Lamictal), valproic acid; the atypical antipsychotics; antidepressants; benzodiazepines; miscellaneous agents, such as calcium channel blockers, verapamil (Calan), clonidine (Catapres); and psychotherapy.

Lithium carbonate (Eskalith, Lithobid) is a mineral that appears to substitute for the sodium ion; thereby, changing processes within the neuron. The pharmacodynamics of lithium shows that decreases in neural activity caused by lithium seem to increase reuptake, decrease release of NE and 5-HT, decrease postsynaptic receptor density, stabilize calcium channels, enhance Ach, interfere with second-messenger signaling systems to achieve normalizing effects, and inhibit enzyme glycogen synthase kinase, and it may have a protective effect on neurons from oxidative stress.

Lithium pharmacokinetics follows accumulation dosing. Lithium is well absorbed with 95% excreted in the urine unchanged. Half the dose is eliminated by kidneys in 18–24 hours; the balance takes 1–2 weeks, with a slow buildup. If sodium (salt) levels are low due to low dietary intake, excessive perspiration, diarrhea or vomiting, the body retains and reabsorbs lithium. Serum levels need to be monitored weekly to biweekly until levels are stabilized and then every three to four months. The agent has a narrow range of safety (0.6–1.2mEq/l); therefore, toxicities can occur in illnesses like the flu. Lithium, an ion exchangeable with sodium, requires attentive monitoring. Changes in dietary sodium intake, hydration, flu status, concurrent medications, and over-the-counter products may alter lithium levels and foster drug interactions, toxicity, and overdose. Lithium has no psychotropic effect in normal, nonbipolar persons.

Lithium side effects include nausea, vomiting, diarrhea, abdominal pain, tremor, lethargy, impaired concentration, dizziness, slurred speech, ataxia, muscle weakness, memory impairment, and weight gain. Long-term lithium use may enlarge the thyroid, produce skin rashes, increase urine output, impair motor activity, diminish creativity, and slow cognitive activity.

—*Anticonvulsants*

Anticonvulsant medications are a useful tool in the management of a variety of mood disorders. Originally used for seizure control in epilepsy, these neuromodulators have found to be active mood stabilizers. The term anticonvulsant is used synonymously with antiepileptic. The medications in this group are classified as central nervous system depressants. Anticonvulsant drugs prevent or minimize the occurrence of seizures. They stabilize nerve cell membranes and suppress the abnormal electric impulses in the cerebral cortex; they do not eliminate the cause of the seizures or provide a cure.

The pharmacodynamics of anticonvulsants comprises diverse mechanism of action influences. There are four main targets of anticonvulsants: sodium ion channels, calcium ion channels, the GABA system and receptor agonist, and glutamate receptor antagonists. This therapeutic classification affects one or more multiple layers in varying degrees by preventing the spread of seizures, depressing the motor cortex and neural discharge, raising the seizure threshold, and altering levels of NE. The proposed methods are blockade of sodium and calcium channels, GABA agonist, and glutamate antagonist. The overall result is decrease in seizure activity by enhancing GABA, dampening glutamate, and prolonging neural firing.

Selected Anticonvulsant Neuromodulators:

- Phenobarbital
- Primidone (Mysoline)
- Phenytoin (Dilantin)
- Benzodiazepines
- Valproic Acid (Depakene)
- Carbamazepine (Tegretol)
- Gabapentin (Neurontin)
- Lamotrigine (Lamictal)
- Pregabalin (Lyrica)
- Topiramate (Topamax)
- Oxcarbazepine (Trileptal)
- Vigabatrin (Sabril)

Sodium channel blockers target sodium channels to prevent the return of these channels to the active state. By stabilizing the inactive form, repetitive firing of axons is prevented. The presynaptic and postsynaptic blockade of sodium channels of the axons causes stabilization of neuronal membranes, blocks and prevents potentiation of the neuronal membranes, limits the development of maximal seizure activity, and reduces the spread of seizures. Carbamazepine (CBZ) is a major first line anticonvulsant neuromodulator. CBZ's main mode of action is to block sodium channels during rapid, repetitive, sustained neuronal firing.

Carbamazepine, as an alternative to lithium, may be better in rapid-cycling bipolar disorder. It is teratogenic; therefore, pregnancies may be of concern. The drug slows communication rate between cells by altering the flow of sodium and calcium. Oxcarbazepine (Trileptal) may be a safer substitute over carbamazepine. Other drugs that act on sodium channels and increase the refractory period are phenytoin, fophenytoin, primidone, oxcarbazepine, zonisamid, and lamotrigine. Some side effects that only appear after a person has been using phenytoin for a number of months or years are overgrowth of the gums (gingival hyperplasia), excessive hair on the face or body, acne, and coarseness of facial features.

Calcium ion channels, like sodium ion channels, are involved in sending electrical messages through the brain. Calcium channels, in particular, are involved in sending a message from one neuron to another by affecting the release of neurotransmitters across the synapse as well as the movement of calcium ions in the receiving neuron. Anticonvulsant neuromodulators target calcium channels and work by blocking these channels. They stop messages from being sent across the synapse either by inhibiting the release of neurotransmitters or by preventing calcium from entering the second neuron. A particular type of calcium channel, T-type channel, is involved in keeping the normal rhythm of brain activity.

GABA is an inhibitory neurotransmitter in the brain that switches messages off. GABA helps chloride ions pass into neurons, which affect the resting membrane potential of the cell and makes it difficult for the neuron to send messages. Anticonvulsant neuromodulators that work on the GABA system receptors are agonists; they increase the switching off of messages by effectively increasing the movement of chloride into cells. Gabapentin works by increasing the production of GABA while sodium valproate and vigabatrin work by decreasing the breakdown of GABA; both result in increased amounts of GABA.

Benzodiazepines, clonazepam (Klonopin), increase the frequency with which the GABA receptors open. Barbiturates such as phenobarbital increase the length of time the receptors are open and, again, affect the movement of GABA. The valproic acid valproates, divalproex (Depakote), and valproic acid (Depakene) nhibit GABA transaminase, the enzyme that breaks down GABA; block GABA reuptake; and increase the inhibitory receptors of GABA. Consequently, they have mood-stabilizing properties. Topiramate (Topamax) is used to control some types of seizures in the treatment of epilepsy. It enhances GABA and inhibits excitatory neurotransmitters. Serious side effects include the risk of blindness, osteoporosis, slow growth, hyperthermia, and kidney stones.

Glutamate is an amino acid and a major excitatory neurotransmitter in the brain. The movement of ions through the cell membrane is facilitated by glutamate. Medications that affect and prevent glutamate uptake (glutamate receptor antagonists) block this movement of ions through the cell membrane. This prevents the spread of messages from one neuron to another. Perampanel (Fycompa) works specifically on glutamate receptors while others work on glutamate receptors and multiple targets.

Anabolic Steroids

Anabolic–androgenic steroids are hormones that increase muscle mass and strength and produce masculinizing effects in the user. These substances either contain the naturally occurring male sex hormone testosterone or are similar to testosterone in their chemical structure. Anabolic steroids are synthetic drugs that are structurally similar to testosterone. The drug mimics this hormone and stimulates the development of male sexual characteristics such as deepening of the voice, beard growth, and muscle mass. This drug stimulates growth in many types of tissues especially in bone and muscle, including the production of red blood cells.

Anabolic steroids are available orally or intramuscular injection. They serve a legitimate purpose when treating people diagnosed with specific diseases. Anabolic steroids are legally prescribed to treat hormone deficiencies, breast cancer in women, hypogonadism and impotence in men, delayed puberty, AIDS, and other diseases that cause loss of muscle mass. HIV and cancer patients, who have lost or are losing their natural amount of lean muscle mass due to their wasting disease, as well as people with hormone imbalance and delayed puberty are good candidates for the proper medical use of anabolic steroids.

Testosterone is the primary androgenic/anabolic hormone in the body of men and women. The forms of injectable testosterone available in the US are testosterone cypionate and testosterone enanthate, both of which maintain blood levels of testosterone for a number of days. Without the cypionate or enanthate "carriers," testosterone is cycled through the body in several hours, so these carriers are important for ease of use as they allow weekly rather than several times per day administrations. Both products come in a 10 ml bottle with 200 mg/ml. Many physicians prescribe anywhere from 200 mg/ every other week to 100 mg/week.

Unlike all the other anabolic steroids, oxandrolone is an oral steroid specifically approved for the treatment of weight loss due to trauma, sepsis, surgery, and other conditions. According to the manufacturer, oxandrolone does not cause liver toxicity. However, there have been reports of people on ritonavir or other protease inhibitors who have experienced increases in their liver enzymes, which made them discontinue oxandrolone. Oxandrolone does not virilize women in low to moderate doses. and it has been used in children.

Anabolic steroids are being used for their muscle-building and performance-enhancing effects, but some current users take these substances mainly to attain a more muscular physical appearance. The Soviet Union was the first country in which steroids were administered to athletic competitors; however, the practice quickly spread to other countries. When the use and abuse of these substances became more widespread and numerous adverse side effects began to emerge, steroids were classified as Schedule III controlled substances in the United States. They were also banned by a variety of national and international athletic organizations.

Anabolic steroids are usually taken in specific patterns and combinations. In the case of cycling, the steroid is taken in alternating on-and-off periods. Cycling can be combined with pyramiding, in which the dose is increased during the early part of the cycle and then is gradually decreased after the peak dose is reached at the midpoint of the cycle. Some users also engage in stacking, which refers to combining two or more steroids (often one that is injected and another that is taken orally). Steroid users frequently practice polypharmacy, in which additional substances (e.g., stimulants or masking agents like diuretics) are taken along with the steroid.

There are a number of adverse side effects of anabolic steroids. Chronic steroid users may exhibit cardiovascular problems such as abnormalities in heart structure and function, high blood pressure, heart attack, and reduced circulating HDL. Other physiological side effects may include renal toxicity, skin and hair problems, severe acne, abnormal development of secondary sex characteristics, disruption of fertility, liver toxicity (particularly with oral steroid use), and risk of stunted growth in young users. Women are vulnerable to significant masculinizing effects of anabolic steroid use. Bodybuilders and athletes often use anabolic steroids to build muscles and improve athletic performance. Using them this way is not legal or safe. Abuse of anabolic steroids has been linked with health problems, including breast growth and shrinking of testicles in men, voice deepening and growth of facial hair in women, and cancer. People who inject the drug are at an increased risk for contracting HIV or AIDS from contaminated needles and lifestyle choices.

Anabolic steroids have also been associated with a variety of psychological side effects. Mood shifts may range from depression to mania. Some individuals suffer from an unusual male body image disorder known as muscle dysmorphia. A behavioral trait is for steroid abusers to become aggressive towards others and have extreme paranoid jealousy. Case reports as well as controlled and naturalistic studies have linked anabolic steroids with heightened irritability and aggressiveness. This manifests, in the most extreme cases, as severe aggressive outbursts known as “roid rage,” which is a dangerous fit of rage and loss of self-control.

A certain percentage of steroid users develop a characteristic pattern of dependence and withdrawal related to these substances. The mechanisms underlying steroid reinforcement are still being studied. Many people become physically and psychologically dependent on anabolic steroids. Steroids are not typically addictive substances, but they can and do become habit forming to the users. People who abuse steroids experience various withdrawal symptoms such as mood swings, fatigue, restlessness, steroid cravings, reduced sex drive, and depression.

Anabolic steroids, including testosterone, are used to treat:

- Anemia
- Breast cancer
- Delayed puberty in boys
- Endometriosis
- Impotence in men
- Osteoporosis
- Weight loss in HIV
- Other conditions involving hormone imbalance

Common negative side effects with testosterone use include:

- Acne and oily skin
- Depression
- Development of breasts in men and shrinking of the testicles
- Enlargement of the heart
- Hair loss
- High cholesterol
- Hypertension
- Increased aggression
- Increased risk of heart attack and stroke
- Insomnia
- Liver disease
- Loss of appetite
- Lower sperm count which can lead to infertility
- Mood swings
- Suicidal thoughts

Positive effects of testosterone use include:

- Decrease in body fat
- Higher energy levels
- Increase in muscle size and strength
- Increased sex drive
- Rise in blood cell count
- Widening of coronary arteries

In women:

- Decreased breast size
- Deeping of voice
- Increased body hair
- Roughening of skin

In men:

- Breast enlargement
- Reduced sperm count
- Shrinkage of testicles

Human Growth Hormone (HGH)

Human Growth Hormone (HGH) is a hormone that stimulates cell growth. It is an anabolic agent that has been used off-label as an antiaging and performance-enhancing substance. It has been banned in sports. HGH can be administered orally or by injection for both children and adults. It is approved in the treatment of children's growth disorders and adult growth hormone deficiency. Studies have shown that growth hormones can help children who are small in stature. Treatment with HGH requires frequent monitoring due to rare and serious side effects.

Dietary supplements sold over-the-counter market themselves as HGH releasers. They usually contain vitamins, minerals, amino acids, herbals, and combinations of other ingredients. One such product is Max-Hgh, which claims to increase muscle strength, reduce fat, improve mental energy and clarity, improve skin texture, aid in the disappearance of wrinkles, enhance sexual desire, restore and strengthen hair length and color, and have healing capabilities. This nutritional supplement, unregulated by the FDA, is not the panacea cure-all it claims. There is no evidence of HGH's claims. HGH is not FDA approved for any of the listed conditions. HGH has many side effects, including nerve, muscle, and joint pain; numbness and tickling skin; carpal tunnel syndrome; headache; and swelling body tissue.

Alpha Omega

Motivation is an important part of any strength training. The dynamics of motivation are simple. It is what truly comes from within one's self. This intrinsic motivator is with us perpetually; it is the inner reason for personal change. Readiness, inspiration, engagement, and retention are all significant predictors of outcome for any change. The ability and willingness tool can make it a game! Honoring the ability to seek information, to become a seeker, and the willingness to surrender to guidance is acknowledgement of the continuum.

INTRINSIC MOTIVATOR

- Tired of being tired?
- Tired of the hustle?
- Tired of the lies and distrust?
- Tired of cycling, spinning, repeating trauma and drama?
- Tired of separateness, having nothing, and feeling empty?

LEVELS

1. Denial (I don't have a problem)
2. Ambivalence (Inconsistent recognition of problem)
3. Extrinsic motivation (Outside influences, " It's his fault I got high today")
4. Intrinsic motivation (Inner reasons for personal change)
5. Readiness for change (Willingness to seek options not related to treatment)
6. Treatment readiness (Acknowledge treatment as the only option for change)—De Leon (1996)

Understanding takes an education. Knowledge takes time to think differently.

Critical Thinking

"I had a friend in high school who was on the football team and was smaller than all of the other boys, and he always got teased for being so. He would always tell me how it made him feel like nothing and how he hated being the way he was. He tried working out and eating healthy to build muscle but nothing seemed to help him get any better. One day, he came to me and told me he was thinking about trying some different drugs to help make him bigger. I looked at him dumbfounded and asked why, and he proceeded to tell me that he'd lost faith, that he tried everything, nothing was working, and the teasing wasn't going away. I told him that it was a really stupid idea because if he wasn't good enough, he wouldn't have made the team to begin with and to ask the coach for some help and advice. He said he would think about it, but I knew he had his mind set on the drugs because they would 'work fast.'

"A few weeks had gone by, and I asked how he was doing, and if he had asked the coach for any help yet, and he replied with "no, I got my friend to get me some growth hormones. He stole them from his dad. I looked at him and just shook my head. I was at loss for words. I told him that before long he would be throwing his life away and that he wouldn't amount to much because that's usually what drugs do to you. He got really offended by this and began to yell and scream at me because I was not being a 'true friend.' Our friendship ended after that argument because I simply did not support his choice at all.

"The season goes by, and I start to notice some changes with his body, but they weren't good changes. Yeah, he did get bigger, but he just looked gross. I could tell he was on drugs just by looking at him. Not long after the season ended, I received a text from him that said he was sorry for what he had said and done to me and that what he chose to do was wrong, not just for him but for his team and the friend who stole it from his dad. I read this text and smiled because I knew that once he saw the wrong in what he was doing, he would be willing to change and do the right thing for his body to gain more muscle and get stronger. I responded to his message and said, 'I am here to help you get better, and I am glad to hear you finally realize what you were doing to yourself and many others.'

"I am still friends with this person to this day, and to this day he thanks me for not giving up on him when he had given up on himself and for not supporting his bad decision because if I had, he says he would have never came out of it because he would have never thought it was wrong. Sometimes it takes losing your best friend to make him better."—Anonymous

WISH

Neuromodulators: Psychoactive Agents

httpswww.youtube.comwatchv=icD3l5bhhKY

Psyche Meds Memorization Tool:

https://www.youtube.com/watch?v=tcwCOrb6LWs

ANTIPSYCHOTICS

Antipsychotic Science:

https://www.youtube.com/watch?v=nGqo7ZQc6Sg

Antipsychotics:

https://www.youtube.com/watch?v=weVoIEWQ9NI

ANTIDEPRESSANTS

Depression Symptoms, Treatment, Causes:

http://thebrain.mcgill.ca/flash/a/a_08/a_08_p/a_08_p_dep/a_08_p_dep.html

How Depression is caused:

https://www.youtube.com/watch?v=KispXWwDaOc

Serotonin Stimulation Medication for Depression:

https://www.youtube.com/watch?v=sr90l6r91cA

Treating Depression is there a Placebo Effect?

https://www.youtube.com/watch?v=Zihdr36WVi4

How Do Antidepressants Work:

https://www.youtube.com/watch?v=G4r3qCkLUDQ

ANTISEIZURE PHARMACOLOGY

Anti-seizure Pharmacology:

https://www.youtube.com/watch?v=tcyBofeAego

ANABOLIC STEROIDS

What are Anabolic Steroids:

https://www.youtube.com/watch?v=foLVCLuVLXc

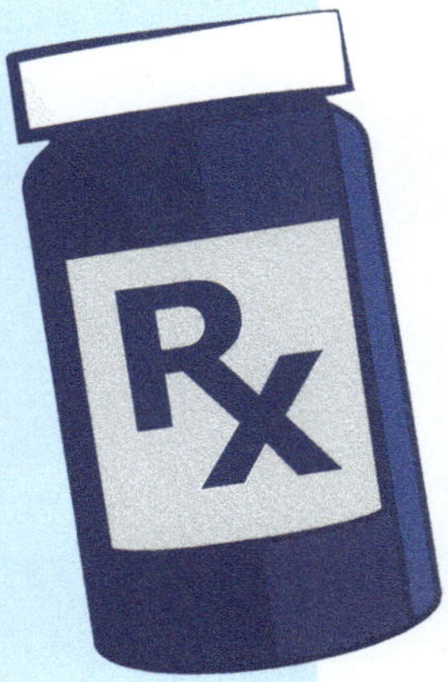

Drug Sandbox

IMPORTANT WORDS TO KNOW!

Neuromodulators
Neuromodulation
Volume Transmission
Antipsychotics
Neuroleptics
Major Tranquilizers
Typical Antipsychotics
Haloperidol (Haldol®),
Perphenazine (Trilafon®)
Chlorpromazine (Thorazine®)
Atypical Antipsychotics
Aripiprazole (Abilify®)
Olanzapine (Zyprexa®)
Quetiapine (Seroquel®)
Ziprasidone (Geodon®)
Risperidone (Risperdal®)
Extrapyramidal Side Effects.
Clozapine (Clozaril®)
Agranulocytosis
Lithium
Positive Symptoms
Negative Symptoms
Neuroleptic Malignant Syndrome
Tardive Dyskinesia
Psychiatric Indications
Nonpsychiatric Indications
Acute Extrapyrimidal Effects
Anticholinergic Side Effects
Minimize Antipsychotic Medications Side Effects with Depression
Selective Serotonin Reuptake Inhibitors (SSRIs)
Fluoxetine (Prozac®)
Sertraline (Zoloft®)
Paroxetine (Paxil®)
Citalopram (Celexa®)
Escitalopram (Lexapro®)
Fluvoxamine (Luvox®)
Venlafaxine (Effexor®)
Dual Action
Duloxetine (Cymbalta®)
Mirtazapine (Remeron®)

Serotonin Syndrome
Withdrawal Symptoms
Tricyclic Antidepressants (Tcas)
Imipramine (Tofranil®)
Amitriptyline (Elavil®)
Clomipramine (Anafranil®)
Desipramine (Norpramin®)
Trimipramine (Surmontil®)
Protryptyline (Vivactil®)
Nortriptyline (Aventil®)
Doxepin (Sinequan®)
Maprotiline (Ludiomil®)
Amoxapine (Asendin®)
Bupropion (Wellbutrin®)(Zyban®)
Monoamine Oxidase (MAO) Inhibitors
Tyramine
Cardiovascular Crisis
Phenelzine (Nardil®)
Selegiline (Deprenyl®)
Tranylcypromine (Parnate®)
Isocarboxazid (Marplan®)
St. John's Wort
SAM-e
Liver Enzyme System Cytochrome P450
Ketamine
Bipolar Disorder
Hypomania
Lithium (Eskalith®, Lithobid®)
Carbamazepine (Tegretol®)
Oxcarbazepine (Trileptal®)
Lamotrigine (Lamictal®)
Valproic Acid
Verapamil (Calan®)
Clonidine (Catapres®)
Accumulation Dosing
Sodium Ion Channels
Calcium Ion Channels
GABA System Receptor Agonist
Glutamate Receptor Antagonists
Carbamazepine (CBZ)
Rapid-Cycling
Phenytoin
Fophenytoin
Primidone
Oxcarbazepine
Zonisamid
Lamotrigine
Calcium Ion Channels
GABA
Gabapentin
Sodium Valproate
Vigabatrin
Benzodiazepines
Clonazepam (Klonopin)
Barbiturates
Phenobarbital
Valproic Acid (Valproates)
Divalproex (Depakote)
Valproic Acid (Depakene)
Topiramate (Topamax)
Glutamate
Glutamate Receptor Antagonists
Perampanel (Fycompa)
Anabolic–Androgenic Steroids
Testosterone Cypionate
Testosterone Enanthate
Oxandrolone
Ritonavir or other Protease
Cycling
Pyramiding
Physiological Side Effects
Psychological Side Effects
Human Growth Hormone (HGH)

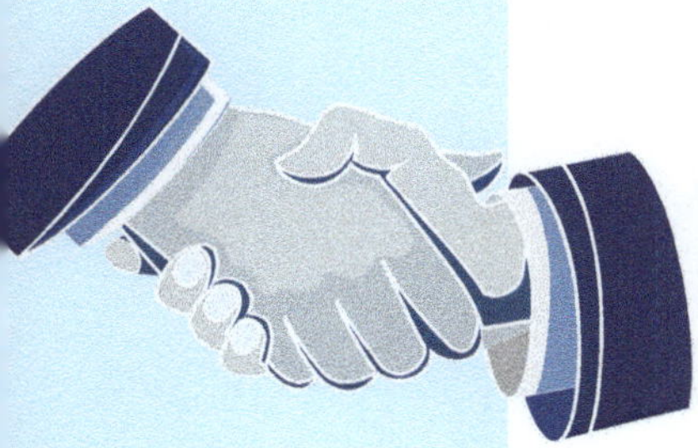

Community Connections

PRINCIPLES OF LifeRing

LifeRing was founded in 2001 and has about 140 face-to-face meetings in 20 states and four countries, as well as online meetings with about 1,000 participants. The program is dedicated to helping people get free and stay free of any substance dependence. LifeRing's website describes the program as "sober, secular and self-directed." "Sobriety" means the complete abstinence from alcohol and drugs. "Secularity" means that the program "supports recovery methods that rely on human efforts rather than on divine intervention." "Self-Help" means that "the key to recovery is the individual's own motivation and effort." LifeRing is a "permanent workshop where individuals can build their own Personal Recovery Plan." It operates as a "strength-based" process that provides positive reinforcement of a member's existing qualities to reinforce the members' inner strivings to stay clean and sober.

LifeRing provides a different perceptional field than AA. It does not differentiate between alcoholism and addiction as it is one in the same. The program does not purport to be the exclusive path to recover from addiction as there are many ways to maintain sobriety, and it need not be the exclusive treatment for its members. There is no one model of recovery that works for all addicts/alcoholics. The program incorporates ideas from cognitive-behavioral, motivational, humanistic, existential, and positive psychology areas. LifeRing relies upon recognized, science-based approaches to treatment. Its secular perspective and emphasis on building upon the addict's recognized strengths and experiences may be a better fit for some individuals.

Demographics of LifeRings' survey of its membership, based on responses from 401 members, indicated: 58% were male, the average age was 47.8 years, more than 80% reported attending some college, and 44% had a bachelor's degree, average length of sobriety was 2.74 years, and 40% attend a religious service of some kind.(LifeRing website)

There are two voices living inside everyone. The primary concept of LifeRing is that all addicts have a "sober self" and an "addict self." It describes the sober self as the part of every addict that naturally seeks sobriety. The "addict side" seeks to control the addict's decision-making process in order to continue using alcohol and/or other, nonmedically prescribed drugs. LifeRing's stated objective is to strengthen the sober self and weaken the addict self by means of providing information, advice, understanding, and encouragement among its members. Members obtain support through "face-to-face" meetings, online meetings, other online resources, and a variety of literature.

People meet to talk about their daily lives, not about the past. Reliving the past is not part of the philosophy. LifeRing is not based on the 12-Step Model; however, it does not consider its approach to be incompatible with 12-Step Recovery Programs and has members who participate in both models of treatment. Unlike AA, LifeRing does not have steps; rather, there are bylaws. It is not necessary to introduce yourself as an alcoholic or addict at LifeRing meetings. The program has no religious basis; it is secular. It does not discourage religion, but it does ask to not bring up any religious views or opinions in meetings.

One of the principal publications the organization offers is its workbook, Sobriety is My Priority. I Don't Drink or Use No Matter What: Recovery by Choice—A Workbook. The instructions indicate that the member is to mark all items that apply to him or her that he or she may want to address as part of his or her recovery. The workbook also suggests that "it makes sense to discuss these issues with a professional." The chapters also include a section for stating a "Plan for Recovery" and a three-month and one-year review to measure progress on the plan.

The alcoholic has the power over his or her own mind and body. He or she makes the decision to not drink. He or she cannot rely on anyone or anything to help him or her not drink. LifeRing teaches people a way of life, not only by talking about the "old days" but by sharing their sober lives and how they deal with problems that come up. By sharing what they do on a daily basis, they are showing those still struggling with the obsession that they do not have to drink. The alcoholic or addict is in charge of his or her own recovery. The behavior has to be changed; abstinence is the only way to stay clean and sober.

LifeRing is open to anyone. It welcomes loved ones of struggling alcoholics and drug addicts. It encourages crosstalk and to speak when a thought is fresh in your mind. In this way, the meeting often turns into a circle of friends sharing their daily lives. It is always there when needed.

End Of Chapter Review Questions

Multiple Choices: Select the best answer from the choices given:

1. SRI side effects may include:
    a. Restlessness
    b. Nausea
    c. Headache
    d. All of the above

2. Which neurotransmitter is affected by SNRIs?
    a. Serotonin
    b. Norepinephrine
    c. Neither
    d. Both

3. Which of the following best describes the mechanism of action of antipsychotics?
    a. Dopamine agonists
    b. Serotonin agonists
    c. Dopamine antagonists
    d. GABA agonists

4. From the list below, identify the typical neuroleptic:
    a. Haloperidol
    b. Trazodone
    c. Diazepam
    d. Lithium

5. From the list below, identify the atypical antipsychotic:
    a. Gabapentin
    b. Chlorpromazine
    c. Olanzapine
    d. Thorazine

6. Negative symptoms of schizophrenia include all of the following except:
    a. Limited speech and emotional expression
    b. Lack of motivation

c. Flat affect
d. Excitation for no apparent reason

7. Positive symptoms of schizophrenia include all of the following except:
   a. Apathy
   b. Hard to talk to
   c. Saying things that make no sense
   d. Not bathing or changing clothes

8. The indications for antipsychotics are:
   a. Antiemetic
   b. Manic episodes
   c. Bipolar
   d. Tourette's syndrome
   e. All of the above

9. Anticholinergic side effects include all of the following except:
   a. Dry mouth
   b. Blurred vision
   c. Slow heart rate (bradycardia)
   d. Urine retention
   e. Constipation
   f. Confusion and memory impairment

10. Acute extrapyramidal effects include all of the following except:
   a. Akathisia
   b. Dystonia
   c. Motor restlessness
   d. Tardive dyskinesia
   e. Sedation

11. SSRIs affect:
   a. Norepinephrine (NE)
   b. Histamine
   c. Acetylcholine (ACH)
   d. Serotonin (5-HT)
   e. All of the above

12. TCAs affect:
    a. Norepinephrine (NE) and serotonin (5-HT)
    b. Histamine and acetylcholine (ACH)
    c. Acetylcholine (ACH) and serotonin (5-HT)
    d. None of the above
    e. All of the above

13. From the list below, identify the TCA:
    a. Doxepin
    b. Quetiapine
    c. Phenelzine
    d. Lamotrigine
    e. Gabapentin

14. Lithium carbonate is a mineral that appears to substitute for the ________ ion; thereby, changing processes within the neuron.
    a. Potassium
    b. Calcium
    c. Sodium
    d. Valproic
    e. Neural

15. All of the following are considered the four main targets of anticonvulsants except:,
    a. Sodium ion channels
    b. Calcium ion channels
    c. Potassium ion channels
    d. The GABA system
    e. Glutamate receptor antagonists

16. From the following list, select the anabolic-androgenic steroid:
    a. Oxandrolone
    b. Oxcarbazepine
    c. Olanzapine
    d. Fluoxetine
    e. Sertraline

17. Serious side effects include the risk of blindness, osteoporosis, slow growth, hyperthermia, and kidney stones from:

a. Trimipramine
b. Topiramate
c. Clonidine
d. HGH
e. Testosterone

Indicate if the following statements are true (A) or false (B):

18. Changes in serotonin metabolism, reuptake and elimination may cause depression.
19. Ketamine appears to be a fast-acting antidepressant in treatment resistant patients; however, it is also an abused substance.
20. St. John's wort and SAM-e are considered natural remedies to treat bipolar disorder.

Applications: Assessment of Usage and Relevance

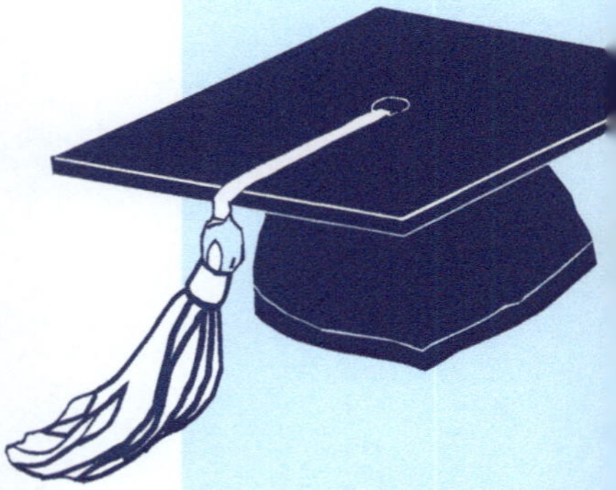

1. John is a 15-year-old teenager who is brought in by his mother because he is withdrawn, has no social life, is failing in school, and sleeps most of the time. His affect is angry and defiant. He is diagnosed with depression.
   a. Select one agent in the TCA (tricyclic antidepressant) class for this patient. Which agent? Rationale why? What dosage? How often? What are the potential side effects? How long until effect?
   b. Select one agent in the SSRI class for this patient. Which agent? Rationale why? What dosage? How often? What are the potential side effects? How long until effect?
   c. The decision is made to give him trazodone. What dosage? How often? What are the potential side effects? Is this a good choice in a 15-year-old boy?
   d. What patient education would you give for TCAs? What special considerations in children?

    e. What patient education would you give for SSRIs? What is serotonin syndrome?

2. Helga tells you she is from Germany and is maintained on St. John's wort for her depression. It is very common in Europe to rely on herbal remedies rather than traditional medicine.
    a. What is the MOA of St. John's wort in treating depression?
    b. What is the efficacy, dosing, and frequency? Can levels be measured?
    c. What are some potential drug interactions of concern?
    d. What are some potential side effects of concern?
    e. What patient education would you attempt to tell Helga?

3. Mrs. Levy is a 68-year-old woman who complains of fatigue, no energy, and no initiative. She says she just wants to sleep all day, and the world seems like a black hole. She is diagnosed with major depression and given a TCA. She is admitted to the ER three days later for an overdose.
    a. What are the signs and symptoms of a TCA overdose? Describe the MOA of what occurs.
    b. How is a TCA overdose treated?
    c. She survives. What other antidepressant would you recommend? Why? What are some special considerations in an older adult?
    d. What patient education would you give her on the new agents? Are there any significant drug interactions?
    e. Why would a MAO inhibitor be inappropriate for this patient? What is a hypertensive crisis associated with MAO inhibitors? How does it occur?

4. Melonie has her ups and downs, but lately her family notices her mood swings are worse. She spends lots of money and then is depressed in her room for days. She is diagnosed with bipolar disorder and put on Lithium 300 mg BID.
    a. Describe the signs and symptoms of bipolar disorder and mania.
    b. What is the mechanism of action of Lithium? What are the potential side effects? How useful are Lithium serum levels? What do they indicate?
    c. Now stable on Lithium, Melonie is put on furosemide for hypertension and fluoxetine for depression. Are these a good choice? Describe the mechanism of the potential problem.
    d. Describe the factors that influence Lithium serum levels.

e. What special considerations must be taken into account in an older person on Lithium? Describe the signs and symptoms of Lithium toxicity.

5. Marvin is a 43-year-old man brought to the ER by the police. He was found in the park dressed in army fatigues, trying to prevent Argentina from undermining the Unites States government. He states that he is a CIA operative and receiving secret communications from a US satellite. He is started on risperidone 2 mg and given haloperidol 1 mg in the ER.
   a. What is an atypical antipsychotic? How does risperidone exert its mechanism of action?
   b. Compare and contrast atypical antipsychotics and phenothiazines.
   c. Discuss side effects of concern. How is this drug and patient to be monitored?
   d. What potential drug interactions exist with his drug regimen, both with the risperidone and haloperidol?
   e. He is now stable and has a grip on reality. What patient education would you give him?

6. Homer has been on thioridazine for several years and is admitted to your facility for alcohol detox. He has a heart valve and is on warfarin 5 mg daily.
   a. What is this drug's mechanism of action? What are the potential side effects?
   b. What are the signs and symptoms of tardive dyskinesia? What is the management? Is it preventable?
   c. What is a drug-free holiday? Why would you institute one? What do you have to monitor?
   d. Describe ESP (Extrapyramidal symptoms). What are they, and how do you get them?
   e. What is significant regarding thioridazine and warfarin? What is agranulocytosis and its significance with thioridazine and this patient?

7. JB is brought to ER. The patient was noted to be smacking his lips and chewing his tongue. He is also coughing up large amounts of greenish, yellow sputum. He exhibits poor eyesight, delusional thinking, and is becoming progressively agitated. His backpack contains cigarettes, a flask of alcohol, and medications: Fluphenazine 20 mg, Benztropine 2 mg,

Propranolol 40 mg, Maalox, Albuterol MDI, Azmacort MDI, and Lithium Carbonate 300 mg; last doses are unknown.

a. List symptoms related to mental status.
b. Is antibiotic therapy warranted? Why or why not?
c. Discuss patient's medication list.
d. This client is admitted to your detox facility. Develop a drug treatment plan for his conditions.

8. Explain the biological or biogenic amine hypothesis of depression. Contrast it with receptor desensitization and serotonin theories.

9. How does receptor desensitization explain the delayed onset of some antidepressants?

10. Describe the various families of drugs used to treat depression. What are the advantages and disadvantages of each?

11. What are the second-generation antidepressants?

12. What are the dual-action antidepressants, and how do they work?

13. What does lithium do? What are the problems associated with its use?

14. Describe, with advantages and disadvantages, the various alternatives to lithium in treatment of bipolar disorder.

15. Describe, with examples of each, the various families of drugs used to treat schizophrenia. What are the extrapyramidal effects of the phenothiazines?

16. Explain the dopamine hypothesis of schizophrenia.

17. Distinguish the positive symptoms of schizophrenia from the negative symptoms.

18. How do phenothiazines affect reproductive processes?

19. What are the dual-action antipsychotics?

KEY

1. D	6. D	11. D	16. A
2. D	7. A	12. A	17. B
3. C	8. E	13. A	18. A
4. A	9. C	14. C	19. A
5. C	10. E	15. C	20. B

REFERENCES

Keltner, N., and Folks, D. Psychotropic Drugs. 4th Edition, Elesvier Mosby. 2005.

www.medicaldictionary.thefreedictionary.com/neuromodulators.

www.news-medicalnet/health/What-is-Neuromodulation.aspx.

"Director's Blog: Antipsychotics: Taking the Long View." NIMH RSS. 13 Mar. 2014. Web. 10 Dec. 2015.

Guzman, F., M.D. (2014). Mechanism of Action of SSRIs [PowerPoint slides]. Retrieved December 7, 2015, from Psychopharmacology Institute website: http://psychopharmacologyinstitute.com/antidepressants/ssris/mechanism-action-ssris/.

Major Depression Among Adults [Fact sheet]. (2013). Retrieved December 7, 2015, from National Institute of Mental Health website: http://www.nimh.nih.gov/health/statistics/prevalence/major-depression-among-adults.shtml.

http://www.emedexpert.com/compare/ssris.shtml.

http://www.drugs.com/pregnancy-catigories.html. Johns Hopkins Bloomberg School of Public Health.

ScienceDaily. ScienceDaily, 15 April 2014. www.sciencedaily.com/releases/2014/04/140415153735.htm.

Hertz-Picciotto, Irva, Ph.D., M.P.H., chief of the Division of Environmental and Occupational Health in the UC Davis Department of Public Health Sciences and a researcher at the UC Davis MIND Institute.

Hadjikhani N. Serotonin, pregnancy and increased autism prevalence: is there a link? Med Hypotheses. 2010 May;74(5):880–3. See more at: http://wp.rxisk.org/autism-awareness-day-antidepressants-in-pregnancy/#sthash.Ym27bhPP.dpuf.

http://www.mayoclinic.org/drugs-supplements/anabolic-steroid-oral-route-parenteral-route/description/drg-20069323.

http://www.mayoclinic.org/drugs-supplements/anabolic-steroid-oral-route-parenteral-route/proper-use/drg-20069323.

http://www.drugs.com/sfx/anadrol-50-side-effects.html.

http://www.drugabuse.gov/publications/drugfacts/anabolic-steroids.

http://www.webmd.com/men/guide/anabolic-steroid-abuse-topic-overview.
http://www.drugs.com/dosage/oxymetholone.html.
http://www.walgreens.com/store/c/maximum-international-max-hgh-human-growth-hormone-enhancer-capsules/ID=prod6181616-product?ext=gooVitamins_ampersand_Supplements_PLA_All_Other_Supplements_prod6181616_pla&adtype=pla&kpid=sku6160796&sst=18c9dbeb-702a-411d-8ddb-37c1267ed7e5&kpid=sku6160796.

Alpha Omega

Vimont, C. (2004). Partnership for a Drug free Kids. (editor) Bennon, C. "New paradigm" addiction Recovery Model takes Lon-Term View. http://www.drugfree.org/join-together/new-paradigm-addiction-recovery-model-takes-long-term-view/.
National Institute on Drug Abuse. Principles of drug addiction treatment: A research-based guide, (3rd Ed.). (2012). https://www.drugabuse.gov/publications/principles-drug-addiction-treatment-research-based-guide-third-edition/drug-addiction-treatment-in-united-states/types-treatment-programs.
http://www.researchgate.net/profile/D_Simpson/publication/13472573_Effects_of_readiness_for_drug_abuse_treatment_on_client_retention_and_assessment_of_process/links/00b4952007121a1acc000000.pdf.

Community Connections

Broadening the Base of Addiction Mutual Help (2012); Published in abridged form in: Kelly, J., and White, W. (2012). "Broadening the Base of Addiction Recovery Mutual Aid," Journal of Groups in Addiction & Recovery, 7(2-4), 82–101. http://www.tandfonline.com/doi/abs/10.1080/1556035X.2012.705646#preview.
LifeRing. Pamphlet, "Choice of Support Groups: It's the Law." http://lifering.org/.
LifeRing, Workbook. http://lifering.org/.
National Institute on Drug Abuse. National Institutes of Health, U.S. Department of Health and Human Services. "Principles of Drug Addiction Treatment: A Research-Based Guide," Research rept. no. NIH Publication No. 12–4180. Washington, DC: GPO, 2012. Print. http://www.drugabuse.gov/.
"Case Study 22: Research on the Effectiveness of Alcoholism Treatment Health Technology." Health Technology—Princeton University 1983: 42–52. Web. 27 Oct. 2015. https://www.princeton.edu/~ota/disk3/1983/8307.

CHAPTER NINE

THE CONTINUUM

Chapter Objectives

1. Differentiate aspects of the perception of desire between attraction or pull and between attachment or connection.
2. Express and apply a code of discernment of choice.
3. Differentiate among the types of neurotransmitters and neurological processes involved with the sensations of love.
4. Distinguish various assumptions and potential consequences.
5. Identify ethical principles and theories of honorable behavior.

Positive Affirmations

> "If we could read the secret history of our enemies, we should find in each man's life sorrow and suffering enough to disarm all hostility."
>
> —Henry Wadsworth Longfellow

Pharmacology

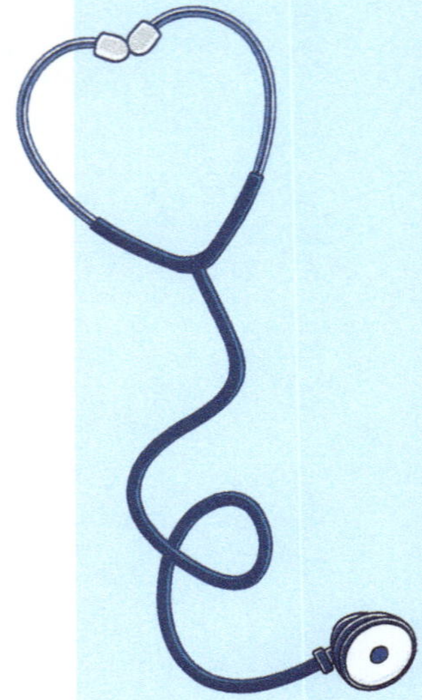

Love

A continuum is something that keeps on going …

Pharmacodynamics of love involves numerous neurotransmitters that play a role in the feelings experienced when one falls in love. Dopamine and oxytocin are two key neurotransmitters, produced and released into the brain, which facilitate the process of seeking, disintegrating, and continuing to love. From the pharmacodynamic perceptual field, each neurotransmitter's action on the brain is either agonistic or antagonistic in relationship with many strategic neurotransmitters.

In situations where particular stimuli are present, neurotransmitters bathe the brain in a love cocktail of stimulating, motivating, exciting, and inspiring substances. Under specific conditions, neurotransmitters are present in large enough quantities and for long enough duration of time to perpetuate feelings of the intense physical and emotional euphoria we have associated with love. This flooding of the brain produces a cascade of neurotransmitters that has been the source and inspiration for countless songs, movies, literary works, political scandals, and acts of violence throughout history and into the present. In order to understand what is truly happening when one is said to be in love, we must be willing to explore these process when the heart appears to take over for the mind.

Dopamine is the neurological component which causes one to feel the initial attraction to something, someone, and some behavior. As dopamine is released into the brain, serotonin levels begin to fall. Serotonin is the neurotransmitter that is responsible for stabilizing and steadying mood, appetite, behaviors, actions, thoughts, etc. This response is individualized. Each experience is personal and unique because the varying concentrations and stimuli combinations have infinite permutations. In general, the outcome reported is diminished appetite, manic moods and disturbing thoughts, thinking of the future, insomnia, and/or generalized mood instability.

Romantic attraction studies have shown that with rising dopamine, serotonin levels can deplete to levels as low as those found in people diagnosed with obsessive-compulsive disorders. Individual infatuation can escalate to feelings of obsession in those with less balanced self-esteem, social support networks, foundational grounding, and dopamine to serotonin ratios. In grounded individuals, for the most part, this influx of dopamine leads to a rush of sensational feelings of excitement, enthusiasm, anticipation, and eagerness to seek out more of the stimuli responsible for the feeling; thereby, initiating the attachment phase of the process in preparation for the next neurological component, oxytocin.

Oxytocin is the connection neurotransmitter. It is associated with our ability as a species to successfully procreate and bear the resulting offspring to ensure our survival as a species. Oxytocin plays an important role in the bonding between mates and between the mother and her infant, as well as in the paternal bonding process. From the evolutionary perspective, love can be viewed as a survival tool, a mechanism that has evolved to promote long-term relationships, mutual defense, and parental support of children, as well as to promote feelings of safety and security. When a woman breastfeeds or spends time in close proximity with her infant, the infant's pheromones trigger the release of oxytocin into the brain.

Oxytocin facilitates feelings of relaxation, reduces anxiety, and, ultimately, stimulates the desire and commitment to the care of the infant child. Without this calming effect on the human nervous system, it is possible to only speculate what the immense stress of infant-care demands place on maternal sleep, nutrition, and parental autonomy. A mother can often sit quietly, watching her newborn infant sleep or suckle for hours without noticing that time has passed at all. The same mechanism of action comes into play when an individual is falling in love.

When presented in conjunction with the euphoric feelings of attraction facilitated by dopamine, oxytocin perpetuates the sense of falling, by causing one to feel the sensations of surrender and desire coupled with the yearning to stay with the source of stimulation for as long as possible. In a romantic context, oxytocin enters both the brain and the bloodstream, leading to the perception of intimacy and trust. Physical and sexual connections with the object of ones' attraction, intensified by interactions leading to orgasm, can cause oxytocin to be released into the bloodstream, perpetuating bonding between partners and increasing the likelihood of establishing a long-term relationship.

In both cases, dopamine and oxytocin are responsible for what is likely to be one of the most intensely pleasurable experiences a human being has in a lifetime. The paradox is that the same mechanisms of action which cause us to fall in love with each other are also the pathway for abuse of substances such as drugs, alcohol, food, and behaviors that can develop into unhealthy, quality-of-life-altering attractions, obsessions, and addictions. It is important to understand how these neurotransmitters affect the body and brain so we can maintain balanced relationships with whatever stimulates this powerful neurological cascade. Awareness, learning to recognize patterns when the euphoria promoted by dopamine may be clouding our rational ability to assess situations, and resisting the temptation to chase that high are crucial to making sure we don't allow out heart to run away with our brain.

Research has determined that surrounding love are consistent stages which can be experienced in variable order: desire, attraction or pull, and attachment or connection, which push our energies to this devotion and passion. Each one catalyzes another, they are all interconnected. In all its complexity, this process is an intimate dance. In the limbic system of the brain, the hormones estrogen and testosterone are activated, initiating desire. The stimulus can be anything, anyone, or any behavior in which we begin to crave or yearn for that sensation of pleasure.

Adrenaline, dopamine, and serotonin concentrations rise, amplifying awareness and sensations. Our bodies react with increasing heart rate, blood pressure, pulse, sweating, dry mouth, butterflies in the stomach, palpitations, dilated pupils, reduced need for sleep, surges of energy, and a sensation of being pulled, attracted to the source. Structurally related substances, oxytocin, the cuddle hormone, and vasopressin, the thirst, yearning hormone, are present when developing a bond, attachment, or connection with anything. Couples in long-term relationships were tested; both men and women had increased levels, usually after an intimate experience, connected with enduring the relationship.

Love, contentment, and serenity are the Divine the ancients sought. The Holy Grail, the Sorcerer's Stone, the Force are all the various expressions that label the love that we all seek. The ancients had several variations; Philiais was seen as a deep, but nonsexual intimacy between close friends and family members; Ludas describes a more playful affection found in fooling around or flirting; Pragma is the mature love that develops between couples and involves actively practicing goodwill, commitment, compromise, and understanding; Agape is a more generalized love, not about exclusivity but about love for all humanity; and Philautia is self-love, which is not selfish. Aristotle discovered that in order to care for others, you need to care for yourself. Eros is the one that causes the most trouble because it is about passion and sexual desire. Unless it turns into Philia and/or Pragma, Eros will burn itself out.

Love is the driver for all stories. What love is depends on where you are in relation and context to it. Security in self-love, self-worth, self-reliance, and self-assurance, which allows us a connection within our daily lives. Our bodies' chemical reactions are a neurological signaling process, a vibration, an energy of heightened awareness to pay attention to! We do have a choice: either to be blinded by the thousands of reflections of the processes choosing the perceptional field that we have no control over, no power, no choice of discernment or to take the time of self-reflection and ask of ourselves is the stimulus anything, anyone, any behavior, toxic or healthy, energy giving or damaging, positive or negative?

In the light of resplendent choice, we have power with anything. There is no greater magic.

αΩ

Alpha Omega

Anonymous ~ This by far has to be one of my very favorite topics, the topic of LOVE. I am, by nature, a hopeless romantic and many times fall in love with the idea of love much more than the actuality of falling in love with that person. I have fallen in and out of "love" so many times; it's much more like an addiction than anything else. Funny thing is, I identify with being an addict, so the idea is not too far off.

There has been activity in a tiny, little factory near the base of the brain called the ventral tegmental area. There has been activity in some cells called the A10 cells, cells that actually make dopamine, a natural stimulant, and spray it to many brain regions. Indeed, this part, the VTA, is part of the brain's reward system. It is way below our cognitive thinking process. It's below our emotions. It is part of what we call the reptilian core of the brain, associated with wanting, with motivation, with focus, and with craving. In fact, it is the same brain region which becomes active when one feels the rush of cocaine.

Like hunger and thirst, it's almost impossible to stamp out. I've come to believe that romantic love is an addiction: a perfectly wonderful addiction when it's going well, and a perfectly horrible addiction when it's going poorly. It has all of the characteristics of addiction. You focus on the person, you obsessively think about him or her, you crave him or her, you distort reality, you are willing to take enormous risks to win this person. It has the three main characteristics of addiction: tolerance, you need to see him or her more, and more, and more; withdrawals; and last, relapse. Romantic love is one of the most addictive substances on the planet.

I know from my own experience of being an addict that being addicted to people is by far the most difficult substance to kick. I was addicted to a person once, and I was unable to quit using him for the highs, the lows, the fighting, and the love. It was addicting. The rush I would receive when things were great, and the low I received when we were apart. It was gut-wrenching some times, and at others, I felt on top of the world. In sobriety, I found this to be difficult to kick as well, seeking comfort and ease when struggling through romantic partners. It is for me to say that love is my biggest addiction.

Critical Thinking

ELECTROCONVULSIVE THERAPY (ECT)—TREATMENT MODALITY

Electroconvulsive therapy has endured a long history of stigma and controversy surrounding it as a modality of treatment. After 60 years of use, electroconvulsive therapy (ECT) is still considered the most controversial of all psychiatric treatments available. Much of the controversy surrounding ECT centers on its effectiveness versus the side effects, the objectivity of ECT experts, and, most recently, an increase in the use of ECT as a quick and easy solution rather than long-term psychotherapy or hospitalization.

ECT is much safer today and is administered in conjunction with anesthesia. Much of the stigma surrounding ECT stems from the early history of using high doses of electricity on patients without the aid of anesthesia. This often led to memory loss, fractured bones, and other serious side effects. Although there are still some side effects associated with ECT, it now utilizes electrical currents given in a controlled setting in order to achieve the most benefit with the fewest possible risks.

Electroconvulsive therapy is a procedure in which a brief application of electric stimulus is used, intentionally triggering a brief seizure. It is not known exactly how or why ECT works or what the electrically stimulated seizure does to the brain. One theory is that it causes changes in brain chemistry that can quickly reverse symptoms of certain mental illnesses. It often works when other treatments have failed. Electroconvulsive therapy can offer rapid and significant improvements in severe symptoms of a number of mental conditions. It is often an effective treatment in people who may be suicidal, and it can be instrumental in halting a prolonged episode of severe mania. ECT is also used in treatment-resistant depression, a severe form of depression that doesn't respond to medications and other treatments. ECT has been effective in alleviating agitation and aggression in people with dementia. It has also been useful in treating catatonic patients as well as patients suffering from extreme psychosis.

Generally, ECT is administered in the morning before breakfast. Prior to the actual treatment, the patient is given a muscle relaxant, and then general anesthesia is administered. In some practices, a mouth guard may be used to protect against damage to the teeth and tongue during the procedure. Additionally, a blood pressure cuff may be placed around the patient's ankle to stop the muscle relaxant medication from entering the foot and affecting those muscles. When the procedure begins, the physician can monitor seizure activity by observing the movement in the foot. Electrodes are then attached to the patient's scalp, and an electric current is applied, causing a brief convulsion, usually lasting less than 60 seconds. The patient remains unaware of the seizure because of the use of anesthetic and muscle relaxant. The only outward indication that the patient is having a seizure may be a rhythmic movement of the patient's foot. Internally, the activity in the patient's brain increases dramatically. A device called an electroencephalogram (EEG) records the electrical activity taking place during the procedure.

During the convulsion, a rapid increase of activity is displayed on the EEG, again, usually lasting less than 60 seconds. The apparatus then returns to dormant, signaling the end of the convulsion. A few minutes later, the effects of the short-acting anesthetic and muscle relaxant begin to wear off. The patient is then taken to a recovery area and monitored for possible complications. The patient slowly awakens, feeling confused and without any memory of events surrounding the treatment. The period of confusion may last anywhere from a few minutes to a few hours or more.

This treatment is typically repeated three times a week for approximately one month. The number of treatments can vary from six to 12, depending on the severity of the patient's symptoms and how rapidly he or she responds to treatment. It is usually recommended that the patient maintain a regimen of medication after the ECT treatments to reduce the chance of relapse.

To optimize the benefits of ECT, it is imperative that the patient's illness be accurately diagnosed and that the possible risks and side effects are carefully weighed against those of alternative treatments. The common risks and side effects associated with ECT generally involve the misuse of equipment, poorly trained staff, incorrect methods of application, persistent memory loss for the patient, and intermittent but persistent post-treatment confusion.

Researchers suggest that this practice should be used only as a last resort due to concerns over memory loss and confusion related to ECT. The effectiveness of ECT is still not completely clear. In some cases, the statistics are extremely favorable, citing 80 percent improvement in severely depressed patients after undergoing ECT treatments. Unfortunately, other studies report that the relapse rate is high even for patients who adhere to a strict medication regiment after ECT. Some researchers insist that there is no definitive proof that ECT is effective for more than four weeks, maximum.

It is not known for certain how ECT helps treat severe depression and other mental illnesses. What is known is that many chemical aspects of brain function are altered during and after brain seizure activity. The repetition of these chemical changes may build upon one another, activating a reduction in the symptoms of severe depression and other debilitating mental illnesses. Even with symptom improvement, patients will still require ongoing treatment with antidepressants or other medications as well as psychological counseling and psychotherapy to prevent relapse.

WISH

This is your Brain on Love:

http://www.radiolab.org/story/91744-this-is-your-brain-on-love/

Drug Sandbox

IMPORTANT WORDS TO KNOW!

Pharmacodynamics of Love
Dopamine
Oxytocin
Desire
Attraction or Pull
Attachment or Connection
Adrenaline
Dopamine
Serotonin
Oxytocin
Vasopressin
Love
Contentment
Serenity
Power With

Community Connections

TOUGH LOVE

"Our mission at Women's Recovery Services is to break the cycle of addiction for women in a safe residential setting, allowing them and their young children to live together while learning the life skills necessary to become strong, responsible contributors in their communities. This is the mission statement of Women's Recovery Services, this is its objective. This program is a valuable asset to society as a whole in helping women rehabilitate as well as learn to be better mothers to their children. Although, at times, some of the program rules and regulations are a little bit ridiculous, it doesn't change the fact that people find and learn useful skills for everyday life.

"First and foremost, Women's Recovery Services is a gender-specific all-women's program. The reason for this being that most women who come from using backgrounds also are addicted to toxic and abusive relationships, and the idea behind this type of treatment is to be able to look at behaviors and patterns without distractions from the opposite sex. This is a smart approach because someone like myself can find almost anything to distract myself when it comes to looking at myself thoroughly, especially the opposite sex. The program has classes daily, and many of them revolve around relationships and how they can and do affect our sobriety. It questions why we stay in toxic and abusive relationships as well as what examples we are setting for our children. Domestic violence is a largely discussed topic in these groups, and. more often than not, the women who are attending WRS come from highly abusive relationships. Seeking safety groups helped me analyze and assess why I sought out and stayed in toxic relationships with men. It was an integral part of my recovery while attending WRS.

"Women's Recovery Services stipulates that there is no nicotine in the facility, the food is portion-controlled, and caffeine and sugar intake are monitored. I think the idea of a no nicotine nonsmoking facility is great. Much better for the young children who, in most cases, were being exposed to secondhand smoke really often. I smoked on and off for years, but I know how difficult that must have been for people who were chronic pack-a-day smokers. Portion control was something that was sort of frustrating for me when I first got there. To be honest, the whole time, I found myself very hungry often and had no options to eat anything. I understand the premise behind this: some people struggle with overeating when they get sober and just exchange food for the drugs.

"It also sets up a routine of three snacks a day as well as three meals. However, never having struggled with weight, I got frustrated with not being able to eat when I wanted and having to wait for "snack time" at 28 years old! Last but not least, was the sugar and caffeine monitoring. This is something WRS takes very seriously even to the point of discharge. Many of the women come into treatment with patterned behaviors. An even though you take the drugs and alcohol away, we still have these behaviors. So, many times, people snuck in extra cups of coffee or extra cookies, and if they were found out, they were generally punished.

"Something I thought was a really great idea was that as soon as you walked through the door, you were assigned a big sister. Someone who shows you the ropes, someone who is responsible for you within the first week you are there, someone who is there to talk to, to explain how everything is done, to sit with during meals, and someone who can be there for you. Going into treatment is scary, especially going into a treatment program as strict as WRS. So it's nice to have as much support as possible. I think that having this type of setup builds a sense of community between the women and promotes bonding. Many women come into treatment untrusting and evasive to relationships with people, and I think this helps them get past that reservation.

"Some of the requirements of being at WRS are having a sponsor and actively working a 12-Step Program, either NA or AA, working with your case manager, following all rules, and doing all your chores. Cold-calling people on meeting phone lists to learn how to reach out to people when you can't get a hold of your immediate support system. Going to all groups and attending meetings. These were huge parts of my recovery this time around. I was able to work all 12-Steps while in treatment and went to 90 meetings in 90 days. I met wonderful women inside of WRS as well as outside of treatment from having to cold call them. I think the fact that WRS makes many of these suggestions early in recovery gives a good foundation for recovery outside those walls. The program helps you get in a routine to live most successfully outside of treatment. I can honestly say that many things I learned from WRS I have taken into my daily life today. However, waking up at 5:45 a.m. without coffee is something I have not!

"I think one of my favorite parts of Women's Recovery Services is the fact these women get to mend themselves and heal their pain all while they are learning to be better mothers to their children. An essential part of the program is the parenting classes that are mandatory to attend every Wednesday. These are a wealth of knowledge, in my opinion. These children have seen and been through so much, and having parents who are skilled with knowledge on how to attend to their hurts and needs is crucial. Also, having children living with their mothers in treatment helps everyone see behaviors and find solutions for the parents and children who are struggling. Parenting is difficult, in and of itself, and dealing with substance abuse and trauma on top of it can be devastating. It is important that we find help to become better parents to our children.

"All and all, I think Women's Recovery Services is a wonderful program. I had a hard time with the 'break you down to build you up' mentality, at times. However, I had to realize that I had to let go of my expectations of what I thought was best since my best thinking had obviously gotten me in the predicament in the first place. I believe life shows up, and we have the option of experiencing it to its full capacity. We can run, we can complain, we can avoid, or we can suit up, show up, and take everything as a lesson to find something of value in all life's situations. Accept that everything we go through has a purpose and every experience we have molds us. This program has been around for 40 years, and I hope that it's around for 40 more."—Anonymous

End Of Chapter Review Questions

1. Continuum: what does this word mean to you?

Applications: Assessment of Usage and Relevance

1. Explain obsessive-compulsive disorder (OCD) and the benefits and problems of drug treatments for it.
2. What role do the actual substances and neurotransmitters play in addictive processes?
3. Explain the three levels and the three factors involved in the biopsychosocial model of drug addiction.
4. What are the DSM-IV criteria for substance dependence and substance abuse? Do behavioral addictions meet the criteria?
5. What cognitive changes may occur in the process of treatment for addiction?
6. Compare and contrast three treatment goals in the treatment of addiction. Which do you think is the best? Why?
7. What are the stages of treatment for addiction?
8. Outline, with explanations, the chronic effects of addiction on body systems.

REFERENCES

Love

Fisher, Helen. "The Brain in Love." Helen Fisher. The Sapling Foundation, Feb. 2006. Web. 05 Dec. 2015.

http://www.youramazingbrain.org/lovesex/sciencelove.htm.

http://www.bbc.co.uk/science/hottopics/love/.

www.theguardian.com/commentsfree.

Portrayal Paradigm

Brain Stimulation Therapies. n.p., n.d. Web. http://www.nimh.nih.gov/health/topics/brain-stimulation-therapies/brain-stimulation-therapies.shtml.

"Electroconvulsive Therapy (ECT)." NIMH RSS. n.p., n.d. Web. 13 Sept. 2015. http://www.nimh.nih.gov/.

"MH Organizations Join Together to #GiveStigmaTheBoot." IS ECT an Option? Mentalhealthamerica.net, n.d. Web. 13 Sept. 2015. http://www.psych.org/.

"Overview of Electroconvulsive Therapy for Adults." n.p., n.d. Web. http://www.uptodate.com/index.

www.ingramcontent.com/pod-product-compliance
Ingram Content Group UK Ltd.
Pitfield, Milton Keynes, MK11 3LW, UK
UKHW052011041026
15590UKWH00008B/2265

9 781516 504145